Girlvana

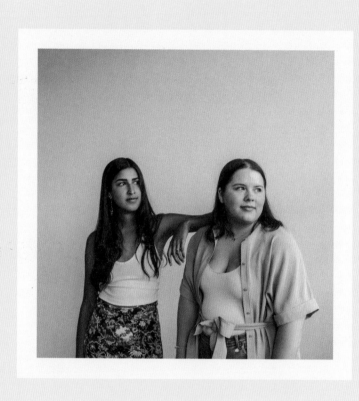

Girlvana

Self-Love, Yoga, and
Making a Better World

A HANDBOOK

ALLY MAZ

appetite
by RANDOM HOUSE

Appetite by Random House® and colophon are registered
trademarks of Penguin Random House LLC.

Library and Archives Canada Cataloguing in Publication
is available upon request.
ISBN: 9780147530660
eBook ISBN: 9780147530677

Cover and interior design: Kate Sinclair
Cover and interior photography: Iri Greco and Jim Fryer
from Brakethrough Media
Photography on pages ii, 80, 97, 98, 120, 179, and 217
by Damaris Riedinger
Photography on pages v, 15, 45, 57, 65, 127, 137, and 211
by Anita Cheung
Photography on pages 87, 230, and 252 by Britney Gill
Interior illustrations: Chloe Devine

Printed and bound in China

Published in Canada by Appetite by Random House®,
a division of Penguin Random House Canada Limited.

www.penguinrandomhouse.ca

10   9   8   7   6   5   4   3   2   1

appetite
by RANDOM HOUSE

Penguin
Random House
Canada

For Great Aunt Dorothy

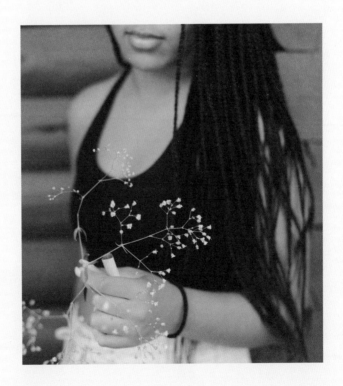

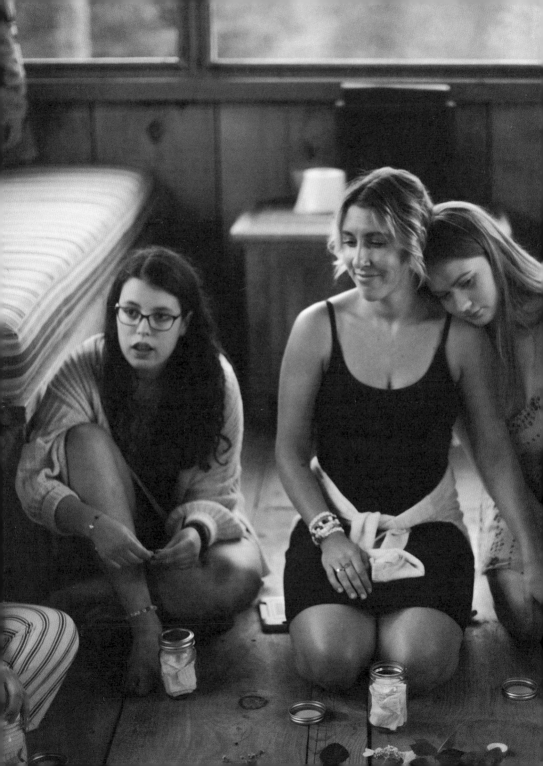

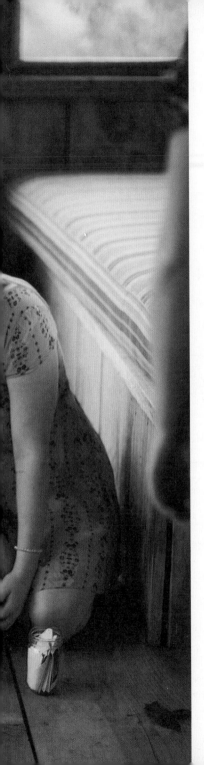

contents

dear girls

dear girls,

This is a book about yoga. But wait—not the bendy-girl, expensive-stretchy-pants-kale-smoothie-consuming kind of yoga; rather, I'm talking about the "Who the hell am I?" and "Do I matter?" and "What am I doing here?" and other earth-shattering inquiries kind of yoga.

Maybe this isn't the way you know yoga and that's okay. For years, I didn't know yoga this way either. I thought yoga was a trendy exercise program for fancy white ladies that drank expensive, organic beverages, that wore white pants and drove white Mercedes. I thought yoga was a parade of thin women walking down the streets of Santa Monica with necks wrapped in wooden beads, speaking loudly about the guru they followed. I knew yoga as something someone else's mom did. I knew yoga as some stern gray-haired lady who appeared as a guest teacher at my dance camp when I was fourteen years old, who kept shouting, "Be quiet!" I knew yoga as balancing on one leg like a tree as a "warm-up" in ninth-grade drama class. I knew yoga as something that was not for a young person like me.

In fact, I didn't know yoga at all. I had no idea what it really was or what it did or that it was destined to change my life. I didn't know yoga because the real yoga hadn't found me yet. The only yoga to be seen at the time was a commoditized product of capitalism that had become an exercise and lifestyle program to "fix you." This yoga was stripped from its origin and true message and made over to fit Western standards. The yoga I was seeing held the same narrative that I had always seen growing up as a teen reading magazines—*This will make you thin and beautiful, be like these women.* Yoga felt like all the other prescribed programs that celebrities touted as a cure to "Reduce cellulite!"; "Beat the bulge!"; or "Drop a dress size in days!"

You see, as a young person coming of age, I had already digested the narratives that society had fed me. *You are broken, you are worthless, and you will never be as thin, gorgeous, or successful as* these *women, but here are hundreds of ways to keep trying.* As I grappled with my own ideas of what it was to be a young woman in the world, society was already shaping my opinions about what was good (thin, pretty, white, clear skin) and what was bad (the opposite of the aforementioned).

I want to be clear that *Girlvana*, the book you're holding now, is so much more. I wrote this book to dismantle the idea that you are unworthy, broken, or unlovable unless you look, perform, and act in the way society tells you to. You are already whole and do not need to be fixed, even if it doesn't always feel that way. This book is meant to unravel the ideas that society has pressed upon us and to encourage a deeper look at how we can define our own value, voice, and purpose in this world. This book is designed to help us unlearn the harmful tales we are told and rebuild ourselves into who we truly are—free from the boxes that we have been placed in.

This book explores yoga through the lens of mental health, body image, relationships, and activism. I will focus more on living yoga versus doing yoga.

I will share with you stories of my own personal struggles as a teenager and twenty-something trying to navigate my place in the world. I will also introduce you to several characters who are inspired by a multitude of female-identifying Girlvana students throughout the years who have struggled like you and I have, but have found their way back to their selves. Each character is an amalgamation of several personal experiences woven together to portray powerful moments in Girlvana's tapestry. My intention, in this book and in all my work, is to provide spaces for us all to feel less alone, less broken, and less afraid. My mission in life is to help us all remember our wholeness and celebrate who we are.

MY STORY

Girlvana is a company I founded at twenty-four years old when I was desperate to heal my hidden, abusive patterns of disordered eating, self-hate, and anxiety.

I can't really remember a time as a teenager when I truly liked myself. I had grown up in a loving family, but I had also grown up believing that in order to be accepted and valued I had to strive to be perfect in every way. I always felt that there was something inherently wrong with me. I wasn't skinny enough or pretty enough. I wasn't popular enough or smart enough. And even though I seemingly fit in as a competitive dancer with lots of friends, I always felt as though I was holding onto a secret. I felt that if anyone were to truly know me, they would realize that I wasn't who they thought I was. I was unlovable, flawed, and unworthy of my friendships, family, and accolades. So I tried to be perfect, and this pressure was painful and all-consuming, like a heavy coat I was always wearing and never able to take off. Was I destined to be a failure, a disappointment, a nobody?

I grew up in what some might view as an unusual household. My father was a famous rock-radio broadcaster in Canada. Every weekday morning, from 6 to 10 a.m., he would broadcast "The Bro Jake Show" to hundreds of thousands of people. When I was fourteen, his face was plastered all over the city on billboards and blown up to fit on the sides of buses—the very same buses most of my classmates took to school. But it wasn't just his face that was on these buses: it was his naked body. Well, technically, it was Burt Reynolds's hairy, naked body (from a nude photograph of him from the 1970s) with my dad's face photoshopped onto it and a big "Rock 101" logo over his crotch. I was mortified that this image was the topic of conversation at school. From walking into classrooms where kids were snickering about what my dad said on the radio to teachers asking for concert tickets or autographs, it was a cloud that hung over my high school existence.

Everyone knew who my dad was and, subsequently, everyone knew who we were. My father always talked about us on his radio show. He would call us live on the air on our birthdays or after big accomplishments. Even pizza delivery guys who would come to the door would recognize my dad's voice and immediately be able to identify him—and the rest of the family, even the dog. One summer while we were on vacation, our house was badly robbed by seniors from my high school. It seemed like no matter what was going on, people knew about our every movement. We were different from my friends' families, who had more "normal" jobs and more "normal" lives. We were definitely a little more rock and roll and louder than your average household.

My mother was and still is one of the most glamorous and gorgeous women you will ever meet. She is an artist, a designer, a chef, and our everything. My brother also remains the most intelligent and charming human in any room, always. He was an award-winning singer, wicked smart and endlessly funny and creative. I'm the youngest, and growing up in a somewhat public way made me feel the pressure to be seen, to be liked, and to achieve a certain amount of success to live up to my family's star quality.

From the ages of three to nineteen I was a dancer—the competitive, jazz, tap, hip-hop, musical-theatre, ballet type. Dance went from a fun hobby as a little kid to a thirty-hour-a-week training schedule by the time I was fourteen. I spent every afternoon and evening, from 3:30 to 8:30, at the dance studio training for ballet exams, dance competitions, and auditions. The studio was the place that shaped a lot of my views about myself and female friendships. I learned that my friends were not only my friends but my competitors. I learned that the skinniest girl was often the most valued. I learned that being sick or injured was meant to be a secret, left unmentioned for fear of being cast out of a show or group. I learned to have a deeply critical eye when it came to my own body and work ethic. I learned that nothing was ever perfect enough. There was always a way to jump higher, smile harder, be thinner, and win more.

Beyond that, I felt like there was no such thing as ever being enough. The constant striving toward some false idea of perfection kept me busy with diets, makeup, and work-out routines. I'd endlessly seek the validation of my parents, my dance teachers, boys, and my friends. It felt like a full-time job, one that I had to balance with school and other important things, like figuring out what the hell I was supposed to do with the rest of my life. I felt out of control, sad, and confused so much of the time, and the only way to feel like I was managing my life was to seek external validation through dance awards, or new outfits, or by being the "good girl" that society tells us we should be.

Now, years later, I can see that I was walking a very fine line of self-abuse. I was abusing my mind with awful thoughts of comparison, criticism, and self-doubt, and sometimes even suicidal fantasies. I was abusing my body by pushing myself to the extreme with dance, training in the studio for over thirty hours each week. At the same time, I was also involved in a very secretive relationship with an eating disorder, bingeing and purging my meals. I was abusing my spirit by depriving myself real compassion and care.

I was constantly juggling the different masks I thought I had to wear. At school, I was determined to be the bubbly popular girl with the best outfits, the most friends, and a certain social status (remaining cool at all costs). At dance, I was obsessed with being the best, forcing my body to its limits to always be in first place. But at home, I'd withdraw, crying, sleeping, or distracting myself in front of the TV and hiding away from my family. Home is where I began to numb myself with food in order to forget what my ballet teacher had said to me or to put off thinking about how behind I was in school. Looking back, I feel extremely privileged that I was able to come home and feel safe and more like myself with my family, but I didn't know how to actually cope with or process what I was going through.

9

THE ART OF BEING "FINE"

I was good at pretending, but the art of always being *fine* was beginning to take its toll, and I didn't know any other way to survive it but what I was doing. Between balancing homework, dance, and friends and the inevitable hormonal and body changes these years bring, I was going through a strange and unpredictable time in my life. No one really teaches you how to be a teenager, do they? You're just expected to know how to harmonize school with work, treat your acne, handle your period cramps, and get straight A's. There's no reference for heartbreak or hooking up at parties or making a decision about where to go to college. All of it is new, confusing, and at moments completely terrifying. For me, those years felt like I was constantly treading water, trying to keep myself from drowning. All I had to do was get through and look good/cool/happy doing it.

There are so many things I wish someone had told me about navigating coming of age as a young woman. I didn't know then that I was powerful or that I had a voice with something to say. I thought my sensitive nature was a curse and that my gut feelings shouldn't be trusted. Then I found yoga.

COMING HOME

I was nineteen years old the first time a yoga class changed me. I had moved from Los Angeles back home to Vancouver after what I deemed a failed attempt at pursuing a professional dance career. I had been struggling in LA, going from audition to audition, being rejected by casting directors. I was feeling embarrassed that I hadn't "made it" yet. My way of coping with this failure and relentless rejection was to binge. I would come home from an audition and eat until I no longer felt the sting of unworthiness. I would eat so that I didn't have to reckon with the thoughts and feelings surrounding my inadequacies as a dancer. After the numbing, my guilt would arrive. Guilt for consuming so much food, food that wasn't part of the suggested diets from all the magazines I was reading. Food that didn't fit the new vegan, gluten-free diets I was seeing pop up in LA. Foods that us dancers were never supposed to touch. And so I would puke. I had trained myself to skillfully regurgitate my over-consumed meals immediately after I ate them.

At that time I didn't see my bingeing and purging as bulimia. To me, it was a secret maintenance that no one needed to know about. It was a level set that I needed to achieve in order to move through my intense feelings. It was a way to cope. I had already spent years ignoring injury and illness, so I was good at also ignoring that this pattern was equally unhealthy. Maintaining thinness and being fine were the priority—pushing through was all I knew.

When I returned home to Vancouver I was sick. I went straight to the emergency room from the airport because I was suffering from a bad case of pneumonia and was having an asthma attack. My lungs were weak, my hair was falling

After years of practicing yoga and walking a spiritual path, I see now that I was a brilliant, all-feeling little force of nature. I just didn't know what to do with that power yet.

out, and my desire to binge and purge was all-consuming. The relentlessness and ignorance of my desire to be perfect had finally caught up to my body. It was time to face myself. I spent months recovering at home with my family until I felt strong enough to move my body again. And when I did, it wasn't through dance but through yoga.

I went to a trendy studio near my house. It carried that same LA vibe of wealth and thinness, with pseudo-spiritual women trickling in and out with their green juices; however, when I entered the space a kind young woman greeted me. She set me up with a trial pass, showed me where to put my mat, and told me to drink lots of water and have fun. She recognized my fear and soothed it with her smile, and made me feel like I was meant to be there. I can't help thinking how different my experience would have been if it weren't for her willingness to show me that I belonged.

I walked into the yoga space and saw something I was used to—a large room with wood floors and a floor-to-ceiling mirror on the wall. However, there was something distinctly different from your typical dance studio. There was a soft and magical energy that felt immediately safe. Music played, lights were dim, and people were quietly moving about in a respectful way. It was a stark contrast to the boisterous and bright dance spaces that were filled with "your competition." Instead of up-and-down looks of judgment on my outfit, body, and ability, I was met with kind eyes and soft smiles.

The instructor entered and met returning students with jovial welcomes and asked the class who was new. I was too afraid to raise my hand and decided it was best to hide. This was new for me, as I was trained to impress the teacher, choreographer, or artist by making a memorable introduction. Instead I hid in the back of the class, terrified about what was to happen next. Over the course of this ninety-minute class we moved our bodies into various shapes and took countless deep breaths. I kept hearing instructions like "Listen to your body, don't force anything, and release the need to be perfect." I had never heard words like that before. They felt extremely counterintuitive to what I had learned about moving my body from dance. Pushing, forcing, and ignoring were a way of life for me. Striving for perfection was the only option I knew. Hearing these permissions in this yoga class felt like a sweet relief. It was as if my body absorbed these words and said, *Finally*.

I felt like I was coming home, to something I already knew but couldn't name. It felt like being reintroduced to myself. Within the first few months of practice, yoga helped me reclaim who I was before my tumultuous teen years. I was able to touch base with the girl who lost her way, and yoga asked me to bring her forward, to stop ignoring her cries and confusion and to finally look at her and comfort her. Before yoga, it was easier to ignore my innermost feelings and to numb my pain and confusion with parties, boys, friends, and dance. I never took the time to sit and ask myself, *How am I actually doing?* Maybe I felt as though

13

it wasn't an option to admit to myself that I wasn't okay. Vulnerability felt unsafe and impossible, and I didn't yet have the tools to untangle my complicated feelings and give them space or validation. What if I unraveled and remained on the floor, a mess of emotions and unable to function? If I felt those scary, buried feelings, would I ever amount to anything? Wouldn't it be best to ignore them and move on? It seemed like that was what everyone else was doing. It certainly felt easier at the time to do so.

Yoga gave me freedom. It presented me with myself, as I was. It revealed to me my wholeness. My okay-ness. My perfectly-imperfectness. Yoga uncovered my years of dark, ugly thoughts and weeded them out one by one. It was showing me the parts of myself that needed my love and attention. It revealed to me how disconnected I had been from my body and my soul. It was teaching me how to love and honor myself. Before yoga, I only knew how to secretly hate, doubt, and insult myself due to the low self-esteem I carried. Yoga was a homecoming and personal revolution within me.

I embarked on my first yoga teacher training at twenty years old, and with that said goodbye to my dance career.

THE BIRTH OF GIRLVANA

Five years after my first yoga class, I began to wonder how different my experiences as a teenager could have been if I'd

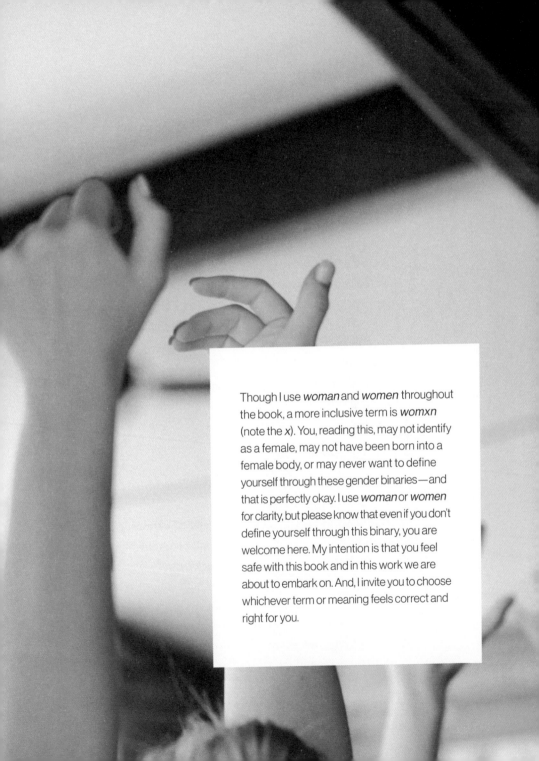

Though I use *woman* and *women* throughout the book, a more inclusive term is *womxn* (note the *x*). You, reading this, may not identify as a female, may not have been born into a female body, or may never want to define yourself through these gender binaries—and that is perfectly okay. I use *woman* or *women* for clarity, but please know that even if you don't define yourself through this binary, you are welcome here. My intention is that you feel safe with this book and in this work we are about to embark on. And, I invite you to choose whichever term or meaning feels correct and right for you.

had access to yoga at a younger age. At this point, I had been teaching yoga for a few years to mostly adults—the same fancy ladies that I had always identified yoga with—and it felt empty. Something was missing. I knew that yoga was helping me, and I knew that if I had come to yoga sooner, perhaps I would have known how to honor, love, and appreciate myself, and maybe I would not have hated and abused myself in the same ways.

I felt a strong pull to liberate and take care of the young person inside of me. I knew that my life's purpose was not being fulfilled by simply teaching people how to touch their toes. I had way more to say, and I knew who I wanted to say it to.

Girlvana came to me in a flash one night. It was all of a sudden very clear—other young women needed the precious tools yoga had given me.

I created Girlvana to uplift, empower, and teach the powerful tools of yoga to teens.

I began to teach yoga to self-identified teen girls in high schools, dance studios, after-school programs, Girl Guides, and anywhere else people would let me in. I would set up in a gross wrestling room in one high school or out on the dirty turf field of another. I felt like a yoga salesperson, lugging copious mismatched yoga mats and a speaker from the parking lot into my makeshift studios. I would lay out the mats and try to set the tone with soft music in the background amidst the noise of high school life. My classes shared spaces with basketball practices, student council meetings, and rowdy cafeteria hangs.

Those early days were really challenging. At that time, the ideas of yoga were seen as religious or cult-like to school administrators, and I was met with a lot of resistance. In those days, there was little talk of mindfulness or mental health in schools. Speaking about mental health was extremely stigmatized, and there wasn't really a language for it yet. I know now that what I was experiencing as a teen was depression and anxiety, but back then I hadn't really heard those words before, let alone known that there were things I could do to help with them.

I had to pitch Girlvana Yoga to principals and PE teachers as simply a fitness class. That was my foot in the door: a stretching and conditioning class to help teens with their sports. There was rarely any mention of the more mental or emotional aspects of the practice. And it was terrifying to walk down the hallways of a high school six years after graduating to bring yoga—of all things—to teens who had no interest in it whatsoever. However, once I had the teens settle into class, on their mats, with soft music playing, I would always begin with a few questions. They sounded like this:

> *"How many of you feel stressed out from balancing school-work, extracurricular activities, homelife, friends, and pressure to know what you're doing after high school?"*

"How many of you feel pressured to act or look a certain way because of what you see on social media?"

"How many of you feel that no matter how hard you try, you will never feel like you are enough?"

With each question, all the hands in the class would go up.

Then I would explain what yoga really was, from my perspective: it wasn't just a tool to stretch, but a way to calm the mind, listen to the heart, and learn to appreciate the bodies we have. This wasn't always so well received. There would be lots of giggles, eye rolls, and uncomfortable moments, but I would keep teaching the poses and slowly the chatter would settle. Near the end of the hour I would flick off one set of fluorescent gym lights and play some soft and gentle music. I could always feel a collective ease taking place. I knew that it was rare for these teens to be offered time during the day to focus on their well-being, and we all need a time to breathe and relax.

As soon as the song ended and the lights were flipped back on, chatter would immediately resume, phones would be back out, and my students would fly off to their next class. I would roll up my cheap, musty mats and collect my things, but without fail, at least one or two girls would linger and then approach me to say thank you and ask questions about where they could do yoga with me again. Over the years, these classes turned into workshops at yoga studios, a yearly yoga retreat on Galiano Island, British Columbia, and finally a yoga studio I co-owned with Jian Pablico called The Distrikt. The Distrikt was created to house Girlvana as well as Jian's youth program, Varsity Initiative. For five years we created an amazing community of young people coming together to move their bodies, express themselves, and feel seen.

I owe the growth of Girlvana to the small spark of interest from a few teens who felt awakened by yoga. They were the ones who wanted to do it again and keep learning more. Those few teens were my hope. The Alexes, the Marleys, the Lisas, the Anisas, the Varshas, the Abbys, and the Emies— the first few whose eyes lit up after practice. They were the seeds from which this book has grown. I am forever grateful for the affirmation of their interest, because it kept me inspired to keep sharing this message.

THE WORLD NEEDS YOU TO BE YOU

Girlvana's name comes from the root word *nirvana*. *Nirvana* comes from Sanskrit, an ancient Indian language, and one of the translations could be interpreted as "freedom from suffering or a deep knowing of peace." As a teen, I didn't know that being free from suffering or being at peace was even possible. I thought that panic attacks in high school hallways were the norm, that gossip and mean-girl behavior meant friendship, and that the only way to be beautiful was to shove my fingers down my throat and puke up my lunch. As Girlvana grew, I began yearning to let young people know that there's another way to experience life, a life in which you actually like yourself and know how to navigate the ups and downs of coming of age. A life in which you can feel empowered and valued and know that you matter.

As I began bringing this program to more and more teens, Girlvana quickly became something bigger, a movement far beyond yoga classes in a high school gym. Within a year it had become a week-long overnight retreat that self-identified teen girls came from all over the world to attend. The retreat was like summer-camp-meets-yoga-retreat-meets-girl-power-rally. During these few days, sixteen teens between the ages of thirteen and nineteen would learn the power of *asana* (the physical movement of yoga), meditation, art projects, hiking in the forest, swimming in the cold ocean, dancing until they were red in the face, and talking—lots of talking. Oh, and crying. So. Much. Crying. The retreat provided a safe place to let it all out, a place where no one had to hold it together. Everyone was free to release the notions of perfection and just *be*—be as we were, share our stories, laugh, move, and cry together. The intention was to be seen, heard, and held by a community of teens and mentors who actually cared. It was—and still is—a time and space to celebrate each other's wholeness.

Almost twenty retreats later, and hundreds of classes and workshops globally with thousands of girls having passed through our programs, it is time to share the magic of Girlvana in book form. I want to share with you what has changed so many young people's lives and has helped me heal in countless ways. I will share personal stories, spiritual concepts, yoga poses, guided meditations, breathing exercises, and journaling prompts in an effort to liberate and inspire you.

Yoga taught me how to peel the mask off my face and the armor off my heart. I know this may seem counterintuitive in today's harsh and unfriendly world. How can opening our hearts and showing vulnerability actually be a way to free us from our pain? Together in these pages we will discover that finding out who we are and what we seek is actually a practice of unlearning, unpacking, and letting go of who we think we are.

21

I wrote this book for you. I do this work for you. It is my mission to be of service to the next generation and do my part in raising the consciousness in young women so that as a collective we all can rise.

When I set out to spread the Girlvana message with my community it started with this statement: *The world needs you to be you.* I still wholeheartedly stand behind this message. We need you—your unique gifts, features, talents, and feelings. We don't need to be carbon copies of who or what society has told us to be. Girlvana is about remembering who we were before the world told us who to be. To reclaim our uniqueness and share it with the world. This is the invitation, and I wrote this book as a guideline to get us there, together.

The world needs you to be you.   *xo ally maz*

01

the power
of curiosity

"At Girlvana I feel loved, wanted, important, and like I can speak my truth."

—Kiyah, 16,
SASKATOON, SASKATCHEWAN

01

ROSE

The first time I met Rose her eyes were downcast, her shoulders forward as if protecting a fragile heart, and she spoke with a barely audible voice. Her black eyeliner was smudged and a constant tic of picking at her chewed up fingernails kept her distracted. She was fifteen, and she told me that her youth worker at school was forcing her to be here. "Here" was a drop-in Girlvana yoga class at The Distrikt, at 4:30 on a Thursday afternoon. The class started the way it always did: I asked a check-in question, then we went around the circle, saying our names and answering the question. Sometimes it was a light question ("Describe your current mood as an emoji"); other times it was deeper, like "What has been the hardest part of your week and why?"

The Girlvana class is filled with self-identified teen girls between the ages of thirteen and nineteen. We're of all shapes and sizes, races, and backgrounds. There is no ideal "fit" for a yoga body at Girlvana; here, everyone belongs. Many of the girls come to this class on a regular basis, and they share of themselves with heart and emotion. Most of them have been here long enough to know that this space is safe to say what they want, so they let it all out. Each sentiment shared is met with a nod of understanding and validation from the other girls in the room.

We finally get to Rose. We have all been Rose before, the new one, the skeptical one, the untrusting one. As the other girls answered my question, Rose rolled her eyes, and when it's her turn, she simply says, "Yoga is stupid, this is stupid."

I thank Rose for speaking her truth and for her candid answer. I'm not offended. I truly want everyone to be able to express themselves and to think critically so I honor the answer and let it be. I then instruct everyone to close their eyes, and I lead us through a deep-breathing exercise. I can feel Rose's eyes on me. I want her to trust me, but I've been doing this for long enough to know that it doesn't work that way. Yoga can feel awkward and scary at the beginning. Closing your eyes can feel unsafe, and I am certain that the "peace and love" language can feel a bit trite, if not nauseating. The last thing I want is for Rose to feel like I'm watching her, or that she has to do it "correctly," so I give her space and focus on guiding the breath for the rest of the group. So many areas in our life demand perfection and playing by the rules—yoga shouldn't be one of those areas, too.

After meditation, we move through the yoga poses. Some of the girls know exactly what to do and how to move their bodies, some take child's pose to rest, and others are on the wrong foot or seem disinterested, but I welcome all of it. We often say at Girlvana, "Come as you are and do what you need." Rose is all over the place, sometimes showing effort and then emphatically giving up. The other girls aren't distracted; everyone continues to move through the class at their own pace. Once we discover how good yoga can feel, or how badly we need it some days, we often won't let anything else get in the way.

As Rose feels her way through the movements, I notice her experience moments of frustration, anger, and embarrassment. It reminds me of my own fear in my first yoga class and my desire to remain hidden. It does feel easier, sometimes, to hide from ourselves and others than it does to reveal ourselves on the yoga mat.

Slowly, with each pose, I begin to pick up on a shift in Rose. Suddenly, there is a subtle willingness coming from her. Ever so slightly, her protective layer is peeling back; the walls around her are releasing into something softer, more curious. I can sense Rose is feeling shaky and confused, but I also know that there is something else happening. This class, yoga, might actually be for her. She might actually feel like she could belong here.

But Rose avoids my eyes. Maybe it's a mix of shame, the need to please me, and a need to rebel and convince me that this is all really stupid. Yoga class is like that—it can feel like we're grasping tightly to our ideas of who we think we are while those same ideas are falling apart and revealing something new at the very same time. I can feel Rose push and pull with liking what she's experiencing in class and hating it. There are moments of ease and moments of confusion and frustration. I feel that way as a teacher sometimes too. It is a lot to witness, this push and pull. It takes a lot of strength to stay the course and let my students move through their own discomfort and struggles, but I know that on the other side of this effort is something really special.

Towards the end of class, we make it onto our backs and a new song from my playlist comes on. Rose looks at me, shocked, and declares, "I love this song!" I smile.

I watch as she closes her eyes and hums to herself. I feel the heaviness she carried into the room begin to disappear. When we arrive at *savasana*, a pose in which we lie on the floor with the lights dimmed and just relax, I see Rose make herself comfortable on her mat as the music slows into a slow ballad. She's made it to the end. I instruct the whole class to take a deep inhale and then to sigh it out. Everyone audibly exhales and settles into their deep, meditative rest. This is often the moment we have all been waiting for, time to ourselves in a darkened, warm room to finally let go of all the stress and tension we have been holding from the day.

Moments later, soft sobs begin to fill the space. I'm not surprised, nor is anyone else in the room. There are tears in most classes. After a long day at school dealing with teachers, friends, assignments, and parents, savasana is a moment of release for a lot of my students.

I look at the resting bodies splayed out on yoga mats, trying to find where the cries are coming from. At first I think it's another girl, but then I realize that it's Rose. Her body shakes as tears spill from shut eyes. No one around her flinches. The other girls know that tears are part of the deal. After a few minutes, Rose stops shaking and begins breathing deeply. She settles into a palpable ease. The room is quiet but alive with energy. Each girl rests and lets the others rest. These girls are all from different schools, backgrounds, races, and stories, and yet here they all are, lying on the floor, letting each other cry and relax.

Eventually I gently instruct everyone to slowly move from the floor to a seated position. We fold our hands at our hearts and bow to ourselves—to our effort, to our surrender, and to the wholeness that exists within all of us.

The teens make their way out of the room at their own pace: back into their phones, back to their friends, the bus, and eventually homework or their after-school jobs. But Rose remains. I sit beside her and ask her how she feels. She looks into my eyes and says, "Better." I know exactly what she means. Her eyes are clear, and she seems a bit more comfortable in her own skin. We both begin to laugh, and she tells me how much she needed that. She hasn't cried in a while, and she doesn't know exactly why she cried on the mat, but she needed to. I tell her I get it. I tell her to come back if she wants to. She says she will and she does, for years.

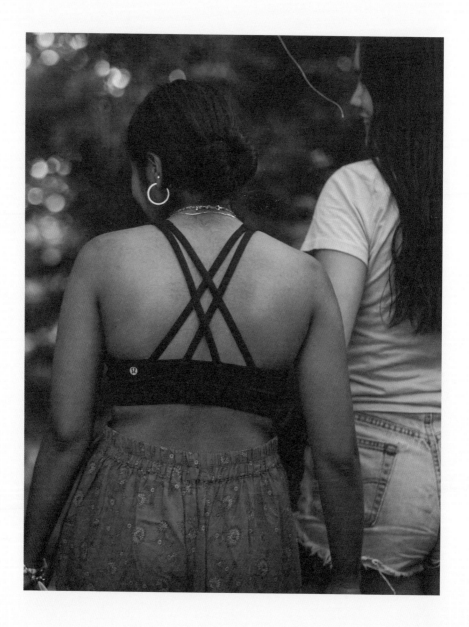

Rose is like most teens who find their way to Girlvana. That first class, they experience a mix of emotions, from "WTF" to genuine curiosity, to a desire to be safe and to be seen. Girlvana is a landing spot outside of the pressure of being a teen, a protected corner for us to explore who we are beyond the confines of other people's expectations. It is a place outside of society's gaze, where we can be exactly who we are and let go of the layers of who we have been told to be.

A QUEST FOR DEEPER MEANING

Before I seriously approached yoga in my late teens, I did take one class when I was about Rose's age. My mom and I went to a community center class. There were six other women, all middle-aged, in the room with us. One gray-haired lady asked, "Is this pose good for losing weight?" The teacher, in a twisted seated pose, replied, "Well, when you twist your torso to one side, you can see how much excess skin and fat is there, and that will motivate you to eat less." Everyone laughed and moved on, but I kept thinking about that exchange. It was the type of banter from women I had heard all my life and come to expect, but I couldn't help feeling that what the teacher was saying was awfully counter-intuitive to what yoga was about . . . even though I knew absolutely nothing about yoga. Yoga *had* to be about more than weight loss and attaining the ideal body type. Even though I was deep in the battle with my own body image, in that moment a seed was planted. If I were ever to become a teacher, I would be one who would never comment on the female body in this way. I'd be a teacher who would welcome all bodies and all beings. One that would focus on the inside, on what really mattered.

I know I look like most of the people in yoga ads and magazines, and I know I look different from Rose and my other Girlvana girls, but I began wondering: How do you guide a yoga class away from the external and into the deeper meaning of the practice? And what *was* this deeper meaning? Surely there had to be one?

YOGA'S ETHICAL CODE
TO LIVING A MEANINGFUL LIFE

Without going too deep into a history lecture, I want to share with you parts of where yoga came from. Yoga's history can be traced back five thousand years, but it's likely much older than that. The first inklings of yoga were found in Sanskrit texts known as the Vedas, written in India. In the classical era of yoga, thousands of years later but still thousands of years ago, there was a sage named Patanjali. He is now known as the father of yoga. He basically took what all the previous scriptures were saying and turned them into clear guidelines on living a meaningful life. He divided this knowledge into an eight-limbed path to liberation that included yoga postures (known as asana, and aspects of meditation, and breathwork, which we will continue to learn about throughout this book). To begin, though, we'll focus on just the first limb—the *yamas*.

THE FIVE YAMAS

Most people know yoga only as a physical practice or an exercise routine to become fit and flexible. This is what the modern-day Western world decided to focus on when yoga was brought to North America from India. Given that Western society is mostly focused on the external and material world, it makes sense that the physical part of yoga has garnered the most attention. Unfortunately, along the way, a lot of the wisdom of yoga has been largely lost or forgotten. I learned about the eight limbs of yoga over a decade ago, and the first limb, the yamas with their five concepts, has been a guiding force in my life.

When I began studying yoga more seriously, I realized that the more I learned about the yamas, the more evidence I had to help me answer the question my fifteen-year-old self had pondered after that community center yoga class: "Is there a deeper meaning to yoga?" The answer is "Yes, there is!" The yamas offer a doorway to this meaning.

The five yamas are essentially a moral code to live by. They provide guidance on how to live a powerful, kind, and truthful life. The idea is that if we use these principles in our day-to-day life, yoga will guide us deeper into our bodies, hearts, and minds. I like to use the yamas as a way to check in when I am feeling disconnected from myself.

Below are the five yamas and a bit about each. Note that these are my own interpretations and are meant to be digestible and relevant for a young person's life. You may develop interpretations that better suit you and your life.

Ahimsa

AHIMSA *is related to nonviolence. This means acting in a way that is nonviolent in words, thoughts, and actions, toward yourself first, then toward others. When you are feeling upset, ask yourself,* Are the thoughts I am thinking kind, or do they cause harm to myself or someone else?

Satya

In Sanskrit, SATYA *means "truth." This yama asks us to get honest with ourselves. Are we lying to ourselves about how we feel or what we think? Are we able to express our voice and opinions in the world, or are we making decisions based on what others want for us? Satya invites you to explore what is real for you.*

Asteya

The word ASTEYA *means "non-stealing." To me, this is about not taking more than I need. This could mean being a conscious consumer: How much are you buying versus what you truly need? Asteya also teaches us to look at who or what could be stealing our time and energy.*

Brahmacharya

BRAHMACHARYA *is defined as the highest and best use of our vital energy. This tenet teaches us to not only look at where we are directing our energy, but also ask why we are doing so. Are you using your energy to nurture external desires or a need for validation? For example, do you need likes or views on social media to feel a sense of worth? Do you find yourself caught up in the need to be popular or to have the right outfit? And if so, how can you balance your energy? One way is to go inward, get to know yourself, and discover what is inside rather than masking it with more "stuff."*

Aparigraha

This last one means "non-attachment." APARIGRAHA *is all about letting go of the outcome of a situation. Think of that old adage "It's about the journey, not the destination." This yama has the same idea. It teaches us to let go of what we can't control and to trust the unknown.*

35

THE YAMAS IN ACTION

The yamas can be a lot to digest, so I have formulated five questions to help you practice connecting with them. These questions can be a powerful framework that you can use to tap into self-inquiry and the true practices of yoga beyond the physical (becoming fit and flexible!) sense. Feel free to use these questions as journaling prompts, or simply go through them now to get a pulse check on how you may already be using them in your day-to-day life.

1. Ahimsa

Are the thoughts you are thinking about yourself today *uplifting* your mental state or *harming* your mental state?

2. Satya

When was the last time you expressed something that felt real and true for you? How did it feel?

3. Asteya

Think about how you consume, whether it's the things you spend your money on or how much Netflix you watch. Are you buying more stuff or wasting more time or money than you need to?

4. Brahmacharya

How much of your time are you spending on the external world? Are you overly focused on what you look like, your social media likes and followers, or having the right clothes? Is there a better way to be using your energy?

5. Aparigraha

What do you need to let go of right now? Perhaps it's a negative thought you have about yourself or the attachment to a bad mark on a test. Can you let go of beating yourself up about something you said?

The yamas are a great starting point in the journey to learn more about yoga, but I like balancing this knowledge with the experience of living as a young woman in today's world.

YOU ARE NOT BROKEN—THE SYSTEM IS

So many teens join Girlvana feeling as though there is something wrong with them—that they are broken and need to be fixed. Many of us have internalized the idea that we are not okay as we are—that we are crazy, weak, or simply "too much." Or that we must look like the models we see on social media and do whatever we can to achieve a certain body type. We're sold so many "fixes": pills to take, diets to follow, and specific ways to act or obey. I absolutely do not subscribe to this idea of a "fix." I believe that what we all need to heal is to be heard, to be seen, and to have a space to breathe—so we can discover that we have always been whole. When we compare ourselves to everyone else just to fit in, we end up feeling weird, different, and even more alone.

Over my years of working with Girlvana girls, I've learned that the messaging we receive as females is incredibly powerful. I grew up feeling like there was no space for me to be messy, wild, or confused, to not have it all together, and I know I'm not alone. So much of our suffering comes from trying to live up to the expectations placed upon us by others, when we should be able to freely accept and become who we truly are. The truth is, the world doesn't make a lot of space for women to feel, to discover, or to simply be, and sometimes it can feel like our only job is to look good and be quiet.

I know so many of us are afraid that we will be unlovable if we're "too much"—too emotional, too smart, too loud, too opinionated. The world has many words for women who are "too much": *slut, bitch, nasty,* or even the dreaded *c*-word. I've always wondered where the equivalent language about men is. Do men have words like *bitch* and *whore* that can be used to describe them? How come when men take charge they are great leaders, but when women do they are labeled bossy? Who created this language? Who built the boxes that we've been told to fit in, stay quiet in, and not complain in? How do we navigate our own identities and our own "enoughness" in a world that tells us to hide our "too muchness"?

These are big questions, and sometimes the world feels uncertain, but I do believe that this generation—your generation!—is waking up and fighting back. A lot of us are bursting out of these boxes. We are questioning the status quo; we are discovering who we are beyond the labels we've been given and reclaiming our power as the unique individuals that we are. We are learning that we are not broken— the system is.

PRIVILEGE, OPPRESSION, AND FEMINISM

As we wake up to the systemic oppression of women, we must also recognize and acknowledge the struggles of Black and Indigenous women and other women of color. Generationally, all women have suffered, but white women have never suffered *because* of the color of their skin. The goal isn't to *deny* the experiences of white women, but rather to remove the blinders of those privileges and become strong allies for women—usually those of color—who have not benefited from the systems in place. Malcolm X described the Black woman as being the most disrespected, unprotected, and neglected person in America. We see a devastating divide, not only in the media with a lack of representation, but also in societal protections for Black and Indigenous women and other people of color, often referred to as BIPOC. This insidious, systemic racism is at work everywhere, from education to health care to political systems. We live in a world that prioritizes whiteness, where white, thin, able-bodied people take up the most space in media, leadership, and politics. So many people do not see themselves represented in the shows they watch, the books they read, or the prominent leaders who guide us.

INTERSECTIONAL FEMINISM

You may have heard the term *intersectional feminism*. Intersectional feminism is the overlapping of identities which include race, class, ethnicity, religion, and sexual orientation. Deeper oppression can occur the more these identities overlap. In 1989, American legal scholar and civil rights activist Kimberlé Crenshaw created the term *intersectionality* to explain how race intersects with gender to produce barriers for Black women. Here is a good example of how racism and discrimination can function together: "A white woman is penalized by her gender but has the advantage of race. A Black woman is disadvantaged by her gender *and* her race. A Latina lesbian experiences discrimination because of her ethnicity, her gender and her sexual orientation" (Alia E. Dastagir, "What Is Intersectional Feminism? A Look at the Term You May Be Hearing a Lot," in *USA Today*, January 19, 2017).

To stand for women's rights, we must stand for *all* women's rights.

I truly believe in the power of yoga and meditation to help us become more conscious and evolved beings. Despite having very deep and ancient roots in India and having been created by people of color, yoga has been sold to us in a way that suggests it is not meant for all people or body types— just those women who are thin, rich, and white. This is not the case. Yoga has been culturally appropriated since the moment it was brought to the West.

40

Cultural appropriation *is defined as the unacknowledged or inappropriate adoption of the customs, practices, or ideas of one people or society by members of another, typically more dominant, people or society.*

We see it everywhere now. Yoga is used as a tool to market health, wellness, fitness, and vacations. The more the industry grows, the less potent the teachings have become and the more mixed up we become about what yoga is actually here to teach us. One of the main reasons I began to teach Girlvana was to take what yoga gave me and to share it with a younger generation so that they could have the tools to navigate coming of age. However, it is important to me to acknowledge where these tools came from and to not eclipse the deep and rich roots of where this practice originated.

I don't want to give you another expensive smoothie recipe or sell you a notion of love and light. Self-exploration is a way to get real—real with ourselves and real with what is actually going on in our world. It's not about attaining more things, like wealth, thinness, or fame; it is about addressing what is going on inside of us and finding ways to make an impact on this world. I see it as a tool to help us to take up space in the world, empower our activism, and take care of ourselves and each other along the way.

BREATHING TO BELONG

My yoga practice helped me understand an idea I hadn't been able to fully grasp up until then: that I belong to myself and also to the world. As a teenager I had felt the exact opposite. I felt like no matter what I did or how much I changed myself, I couldn't feel the safety of belonging. Even though I faked it and from the outside it looked as though I fit in, deep down, I felt differently. I felt fragmented, and disconnected from my body and my emotions. It felt as though I was ruled by my constant overthinking and self-criticism. I felt so uncomfortable in my body and existing as "me"— whoever that was. So, to deal with that uncomfortable feeling, I would search for something to make it better, or different, often by buying something, bingeing and purging, or seeking validation from others, but at the end of the day I was stuck in this constant cycle of *blah*. I was certain that nobody else felt this way and the thought of sharing how I felt was a huge impossibility. As if I was going to casually mention to my mom or at a sleepover with friends that being me was the most terrible and terrifying experience. It was easier to just be fine. You know how it goes:

How are you?

Fine.

I believed that if I actually expressed all the dark thoughts I was having, no one would care. So I locked it up like a secret and felt destined to always feel this way.

One of the first things you learn in yoga is how to breathe properly. When I was taught the power of breath, it was as though something came back to me, a freedom, a place to exist. It was as if a sense of belonging had been alive inside of me the whole time, just waiting to be discovered.

The practice of breathing deeply with focused attention helps you to regulate your thoughts and dissolve anxiety. When you breathe in, or inhale, you draw fresh oxygen into the brain and bloodstream, which has an energizing and clarifying effect on the nervous system. When you breathe out, exhale, you release carbon dioxide (CO_2) and toxins, creating a soothing and calming effect on the body, mind, and emotions.

Through yoga, I learned that breath was a way for me to shift the experience of the disconnection I was feeling within. When I learned how to breathe deeply, I began to experience a sense of ease and comfort within myself that I previously had not known. And it didn't cost anything! I could do it anywhere, whenever I needed to, and it was my way to immediately pull myself into the present moment. So many people don't know about the power of breath! In every moment this gift is available, and yet so many of us don't realize it or have simply forgotten.

HOW TO BREATHE

The simplest visual for the breath is to imagine that a balloon is being blown up and then slowly deflated.

1. Place one hand on your chest and the other hand on your belly.

2. Take a deep inhale through your nose. Feel your lungs and belly expand. Visualize your belly expanding with air like a balloon.

3. Exhale through your nose or mouth as slowly as you can. Imagine the balloon slowly deflating. Feel your belly button draw back toward your spine.

4. Try to count four beats as you inhale and four beats as you exhale. *Inhale, two, three, four. Exhale, two, three, four.*

5. Repeat for ten breath cycles.

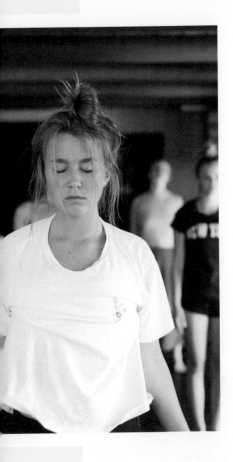

It is important to note that training the body to breathe like this takes time, which is why practice is so important. When we aren't breathing to full capacity, we may feel more fatigued or distracted. It is important to breathe as deeply as we can to energize and oxygenate ourselves.

Check on yourself right now. Does your breath feel shallow and tight? Does your breath feel calming and nourishing? There is no right or wrong answer here; what is important is that you be present as you breathe in and out. The more we focus on the breath, the deeper it will become. There is no rush to perfect it. It is simply a practice of focusing on the inhale and exhale until we start to feel a sense of calm.

In today's world, we are constantly being pulled out of the present moment— by our devices or by our constantly overthinking minds. In these moments, breath is your greatest tool. Treat it as the ultimate reset.

45

PRESENT-MOMENT AWARENESS

Let's look at the breath a little more deeply now by really paying attention to what is going on as you breathe. No need to judge yourself; just be mindful.

46

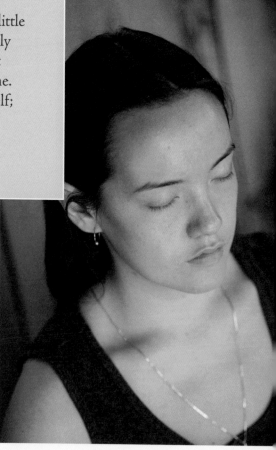

1. Become aware of your breath. There's no need to change it in any way; just notice if it's shallow or tight anywhere in your body. Where do you feel it in your body? Do your lungs or belly expand when you inhale or does the breath feel trapped in your throat and shoulders?

2. Begin to deepen your inhale by taking a longer breath in through your nose. Feel your chest and belly inflate like a balloon being blown up. Let the belly and chest really enlarge and expand. Gently pause at the top of the breath when you feel like you can't inhale anymore.

3. Exhale through your nose or mouth as slowly as you can, letting your mind follow the breath out. As you do this, relax your shoulders and your jaw. Let your belly relax like a balloon losing its air.

4. Repeat at least five times, in and out, trying to keep your mind focused on your breath. Don't worry if you lose focus; that is perfectly normal. Use the next inhale as a reset to try again.

47

After five rounds, notice how you feel. Notice what you see. Notice if there is a feeling of more space inside your mind or body. You may notice that you feel calmer and more open. This kind of breathing exercise takes some getting used to, but the more we practice mindfully breathing, the easier it comes and the better we feel.

WHO THE HELL AM I?

Now that we have been introduced to a few fundamentals of yoga and have a good idea of what elongating and deepening our breath feels like, I want to take a deep dive into the heart of the matter. It's nice to conceptualize a few yogic ideas and to feel our breath, but self-inquiry is another part of yoga.

Who the hell am I? This is the question I hear the most as a yoga teacher to teens. It's also the question I most often ask myself, an adult woman, and that all of us ask ourselves in our lifetimes. It is a spiritual question and one of the deepest inquiries there is. It often shows up at the beginning of spiritual quests, and this is why I present it to you here in the first chapter. It is important. You are important. So together, let's begin this journey.

WHO AM I?

When we are teenagers, we are seeking out our identity and trying to define ourselves. We can straddle this fine line of wanting to fit in while also needing to stand out, as well as feeling young but having to start thinking about more adult things. We may look for things that define us, like friend groups, music, fashion, academics, or sports, because it feels safe and it makes us feel like we belong. There is absolutely nothing wrong with that. Who you hang out with and what you do are of course important, but it's also important that you know who you are without these things. That's how you truly learn who you are.

If I were to ask you right now "Who are you?" how would you answer? When I was a teen my first response would have been "a dancer." I thought the thing that I *did* was who I *was*. We all do this. We define ourselves through what we do, what we wear, and what we have. A few years after high school I stopped dancing, and I felt so lost because I thought I had lost the essence of who I was.

I've experienced this when romantic relationships have ended, too, as well as when I've lost or grown out of friendships. After my first relationship ended, I was heartbroken and I had no idea who I was. My identity had been so wrapped up in the person I was dating, I couldn't see the rest of my life, and everything I *did* have.

I see spirituality as knowing who you are without the things that define you. Yes, I am a yoga teacher, a wife, a mentor, and a writer—but without those things, I am still me. Even if I didn't have any of these roles, I still have value and worth in this world.

That doesn't mean I love those roles any less, that being a yoga teacher or wife isn't important to me; it just means that there is more to me beyond them, the people I hang out with, or the work that I do. Life is ever changing, and circumstances and people will inevitably shift. We can prepare ourselves for life by identifying with who we *are* versus what we have or do.

YOUR "I AM" STATEMENT

So who are you? Let's continue to unpack this. Grab your pen and journal and write down the following:

What do I do?
    List schoolwork, your job, activities, hobbies, sports, extracurriculars—all the things that you spend your time doing.

Who do I know?
    List your relationships, friend groups, family, clubs, your partner if you have one. This is your network.

What do I have?
    List the material things that are important to you, like clothes, brands, devices, awards, and even grades.

Who am I without those things?
    Take a minute to think about this, and then list who you are without what you do, who you know, and what you have. Dig deep here. You may feel sad, devastated, or lost without the things that define you, but I want you to look at who you are without them as a way to see that *you are still you.* You are still kind, smart, funny, compassionate,

and caring. When I'm reflecting on who I am without the things and labels I've given myself (or that have been given to me), I sometimes will think about who I was as a young child. Try it: What qualities did you possess before you wrapped yourself up in someone or something else? One of my favorite questions to ask is, *Who were you before the world told you who to be?*

Now, the big question: Who am I?
Reiterate who you are in a clearer way. Are you resilient, joyful, open-minded? Are you intelligent, curious, passionate, and brave? Who you are should have nothing to do with the clothes you wear or the people you hang out with; it's about who you are *inside*. Search for the essence of yourself here, that which is unshakable and that no one can take away from you.

51

You see, when we are attached to things and people and those things disappear, we think *we* disappear. But we don't. I can't tell you how many times I thought I would die of heartbreak or that I would not survive after a friend had walked away from me. I suffered immensely because I thought that the person I loved was a *part* of me, that I needed them to survive. But that wasn't true. What I didn't know back then was that when endings come, which they inevitably will, we can survive as we are. We can even thrive when we know who we are without these things that have previously defined us.

Who were you before the world told you who to be?

I find that when I appreciate what I have and who I have in my life without attaching my identity to it or them, I can appreciate what I have and not be defined by it.

Without these things, we are still us. So, who are you? Below are some words to inspire you:

Powerful	*Joyful*	*Resilient*	*Audacious*
Brave	*Free*	*Strong*	*Sincere*
Smart	*Passionate*	*Fierce*	*Authentic*
Loving	*Radiant*	*Compassionate*	
Adventurous	*Kind*	*Empathetic*	

DECLARE YOURSELF

Create an "I am" statement pulling from the words that you discovered about yourself that describe you are beyond what you do or who you spend your time with. This could be as simple as writing it down on a sticky note or as fancy as a huge, bedazzled poster board. You get to choose how and where this statement shows up in your life.

Here's an example:

I am fearlessly loving.
I am expressive and creative.
I am worthy without anything defining me.

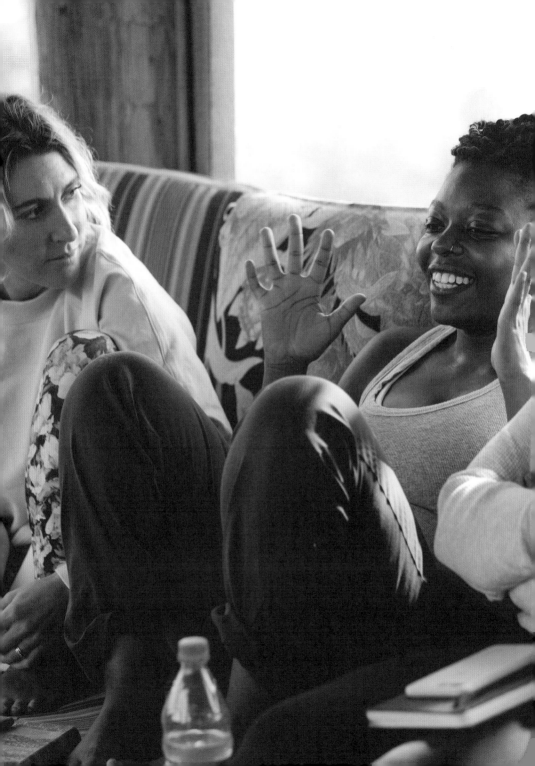

I love keeping "I am" statements around my house and scribbled into my notebook. They serve as reminders when I get caught up in my work and in my personal life. When I am suffering from a disappointment or a situation that I cannot control, I can come back to my "I am" and remember I am more than what I am currently going through or how people have defined me.

I invite you to post your "I am" statement in your room, bathroom, locker, mirror, or wallet and look at it as many times throughout the day as you need. It is important to know that regardless of what or who leaves, disappears, fails, or dissolves from your life, *you are still you.* You still belong to yourself. You still have a place in this world.

INTRO TO MEDITATION

I used to think that there was a "right" way to meditate and that if I tried, I would just get it wrong. Many of us assume that meditation looks something like this: we sit down and close our eyes, and all of our thoughts disappear. Well, that simply is not true. Yes, you sit down, but you can also lie down or be in any other position that makes you feel comfortable. You can close your eyes, but you can also soften your gaze if you are not comfortable with closing your eyes just yet. And no, the thoughts don't just disappear! It takes practice for the mind to slow down and not be all over the place. I think this is why meditating can be so intimidating—because our thoughts can seem so loud. I am here to tell you that it is normal and totally fine to be thinking while you are meditating.

YOUR MIND IS A PUPPY

I like the analogy of seeing the mind as an adorable little puppy that can't sit still. It wanders away with any small distraction, and you have to continue to call it back and say, "Sit" or "Stay." I like this puppy analogy because it keeps me compassionate and tender towards my chaotic thoughts. (And who doesn't love puppies?!) Instead of being harsh toward myself for thinking too much, I just think about that little puppy. Instead of punishing or abandoning it, I tell it to come back to me. The puppy is something I want to take care of and nourish. Seeing the mind this way, as something to be taken care of and paid attention to, can support our mental health greatly.

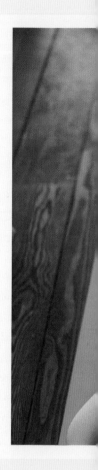

HOW TO MEDITATE

I'd like to introduce you to a really simple way to meditate.

1. Get comfortable, whether that is by sitting or by lying down.

2. Close your eyes or let your gaze fix on one thing.

3. Inhale and silently repeat, *I am breathing in.*

4. Exhale and silently repeat, *I am breathing out.*

5. Repeat this ten times.

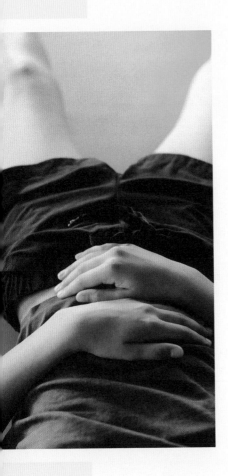

As you are first learning to meditate, it can be helpful to set a timer for three minutes and begin to build your time up from there. Once you've finished the exercise, notice how you feel. Did anything change in your body, mind, or heart? How do you feel after you take this time? Remember, if your puppy mind wandered away during this meditation, that's perfectly normal. I find that using the words *I am breathing in* and *I am breathing out* is a good way to come back to the present moment.

This exercise is a simple way to start a meditation practice, and it can be done anywhere and anytime you like. Meditation doesn't have to be a fancy, unattainable thing. It can be yours to explore and define for yourself. I encourage you to keep trying and see what you discover about the way meditation makes you feel. Use the puppy-dog analogy if it helps. Training our minds with patience and forgiveness is essential in this process.

THE "I AM" MEDITATION

Keeping the above meditation as
a base, we can begin to move on
to another powerful meditation,
called "I Am." I like using this
meditation when I'm beginning
to lose sight of who I am or when
I feel lost in someone or something
else. This is a powerful way to
remember who we are and break
the trance of negative thoughts
we have about ourselves.

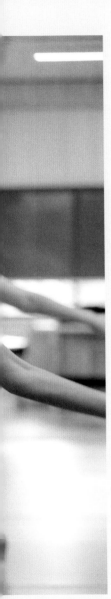

1. Get comfortable and close your eyes or soften your gaze. Become aware of your inhale and exhale and begin to deepen the breath.

2. As you inhale, begin imagining that you are limitless. There are no boundaries or expectations, just pure possibility.

3. As you exhale, imagine letting go of any false ideas that you or anyone else holds of you. Release old versions of yourself. Let go of who you think you have to be.

4. Repeat this cycle five times with the intention of letting go. Inhale *possibility* and exhale releasing *expectations*.

5. Keeping your gaze soft or eyes closed, focus on the "I am" statement that you created earlier (page 50).

6. Connect your inhale to the words *I am*.

7. Connect your exhale to the end of that statement.

8. Inhale *I am*, exhale your word.

9. Repeat your "I am" statement ten times.

59

When we repeat our "I am" statement in meditation like this, it can help us truly believe these words. I encourage you to practice repeating your personal statement often and note any changes that this practice is making within your life.

FINDING YOUR DAILY SADHANA

One of the ways we can continue to discover who we are is by having a daily practice. In yoga we call this *sadhana*. To remember how to spell this Sanskrit word, some of my students call it Sad Hana. What do we do when Hana is sad? Practice, of course!

Sadhana is the personal, spiritual effort you can tap into as a daily practice to find more peace and well-being. Only you get to define what that means for you. Think of it as a way to feel more grounded and connected to yourself. It is also a way to set yourself up before the busyness and chaos of our days begin. Sometimes we try to establish big, lofty goals that end up falling away in a short amount of time because they are unsustainable, like trying to tick off everything on our to-do lists and overextending ourselves when we are feeling tired. Your sadhana is meant to sustain your well-being, so when you're developing your own, choose practices that fulfill you, reset you, and most importantly feel doable.

Here are a few examples:
+ making a cup of tea in the morning and enjoying it without looking at your phone
+ listening to your favorite music as you walk to school
+ taking time to journal in the morning
+ doing your sun salutations (page 67)
+ saying a prayer
+ doing your meditation for empowerment

The important thing to keep in mind when creating your own sadhana is not *what* you are doing, but *why* you are doing it. For me having a sadhana is essential for my well-being. It is a commitment to myself. Another name for sadhana is *ritual*. What are a few practices you can find each day that support you?

A personal practice is important because it breaks up our negative habitual patterns. In yoga we call these *samskaras*. Samskaras are said to be energetic impressions or grooves set into in the mind that create habits. The stronger the habit is, the harder it is to break and choose something different. We often don't know that we are operating from an unconscious, habitual place. This can look like a cycle of negative thoughts and feelings constantly circulating in the mind and bringing you down. When we begin a daily practice, we are creating a healthy habit, and we begin to rewire our default negative mental state.

If I could guess what our generation's morning habit would be, I'd guess checking our phones the moment we wake up. I am guilty of this myself, even though I know that seeing other people's seemingly perfect lives can immediately make me feel bad, especially if I'm struggling in my life at that moment. When I commit to breathing deeply, saying my "I am" statement, or meditating in the morning, I am more inclined to keep my day on track with positive habits. My sadhana grounds me before the outside world can make its impression on me.

By keeping your sadhana small and sacred, you will be able to find pockets of peace throughout your day. I encourage you to find one small habit (remember, something small and doable; nothing too lofty and thus hard to keep going) that you can define as sadhana for seven days. You can journal about this small moment and how it affects you from day to day, and hopefully over time, these tiny rituals will make up a spiritual practice that is unique and fulfilling to you.

BODY, MIND, HEART, SOUL

Throughout this book, you will see how the weaving together of our bodies, minds, hearts, and souls is essential to our well-being. The yoga asana (postures) give us the opportunity to bridge these four pillars. We will continuously explore the ways in which we can support all four of these places within us.

When we move our bodies and use our breath, our minds can become clearer, our hearts can become more open, and our souls can speak. Moving our bodies with yoga asana is healthy not only for the physical body but also for our mental, emotional, and spiritual health.

YOGA ASANA

Yoga asana, the postures or poses, are an amazing way to move our bodies. And guess what? You don't have to be flexible or strong to start a physical yoga practice. That is why it's called a practice. It is something to learn and get better at with time, not something you have to already know and need to perfect. That's one of the reasons I love yoga.

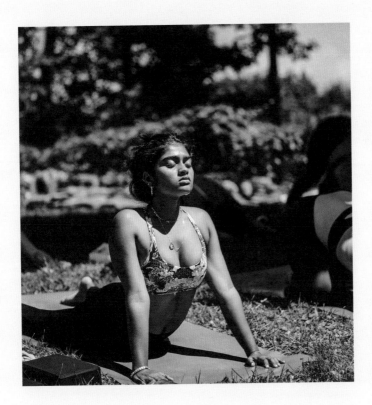

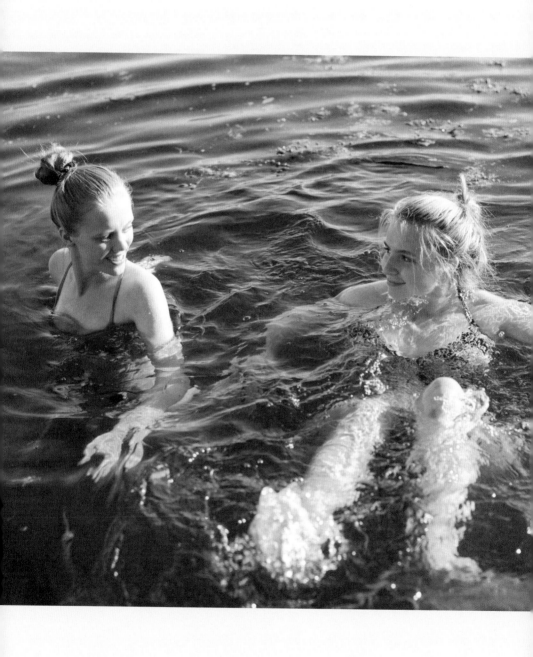

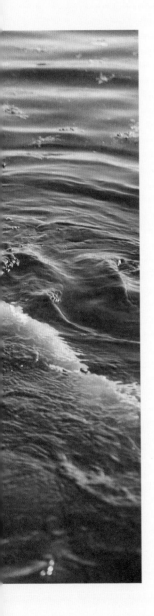

A PRACTICE IN FLUIDITY

Forget about fancy studio memberships or even having a yoga mat. The sun salutation is a simple routine that is the basis of a yoga flow, and you can do it anywhere. Sun salutations offer a ton of benefits, including getting the blood moving, bringing oxygen into your brain, energizing you, and creating mental clarity. They also stretch and strengthen the body. The aim of yoga is to create union and help balance us out mentally, physically, and emotionally. When these pillars come together in harmony it can feel like a spiritual experience for your soul.

Try the asana sequence on the following page three times and notice how you feel afterward. Don't let a lack of time or space deter you—you only need a little bit of room and a few minutes. A little movement goes a really long way!

65

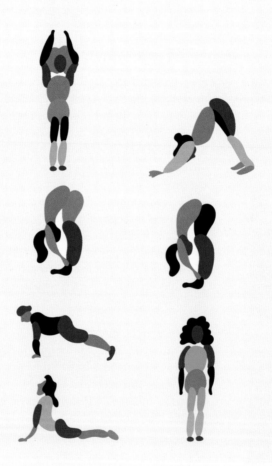

SUN SALUTATIONS

1. Stand tall with your feet hip-distance apart, arms by your side.

2. Inhale and lift your arms over your head.

3. Exhale and fold over your legs in a forward bend. Bend your knees if you need to.

4. Inhale and step back into a plank position. You can drop your knees if you need to.

5. Exhale, bend your elbows, and come to lay your whole body on the floor.

6. Press into your hands and lift your chest up off the ground any amount. This is cobra pose.

7. Exhale, tuck your toes, and come into downward dog—an upside-down V shape.

8. Step forward and into another forward bend.

9. Inhale, reaching your arms up over your head.

10. Exhale, fold back over your legs, and repeat.

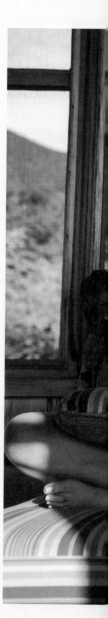

JOURNAL

Journaling plays a big role in Girlvana. It's another avenue of expression. Sometimes we express ourselves through movement or talking, and other times it feels better to just write it all down. So, at the end of each chapter, there will be a journaling prompt that will help you to reflect on what we've talked about in the chapter.

We've spent this chapter exploring the idea of who we are and what roles we play, and we've just begun to investigate the ways in which we have been told to act and behave in this world. The question on the next page allows us to discover and reclaim who we are beyond the conditioning we have received as girls. The question is meant to stir up any ideas of who we think we should be and steer us back to the person we truly are.

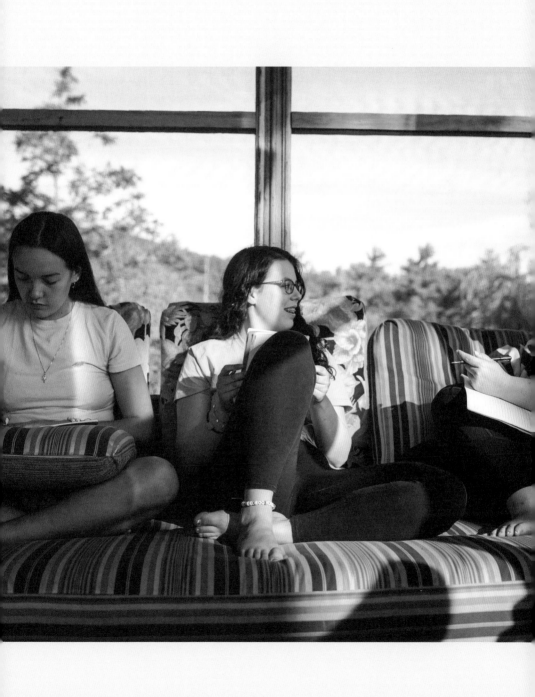

Who were you before the world told you who to be?

I love this question because it allows us to dig into who we are beyond the societal norms. It makes us remember who we were as children and connects us to a time where what we had and who we knew did not define us. It was more about play and finding joy. It was about being who we were without fear. I encourage you to remember who that was as it is a way to know who you currently are.

YOUR TURN.

_____

_____

_____

_____

_____

_____

_____

_____

_____

_____

_____

If you ever feel like you simply cannot go on, access to therapy or a school counselor can be vital. Yoga has always been there for me. So has therapy. There is absolutely nothing wrong with seeking help.

02

the power of
your body

"Home is not just the place where you get up every morning and come home every night. I have found a new home in the shelter of my body, one which I had rejected previously."

—Flic, 15,
BATH, ENGLAND

02

SHERICE

Everyone arrived by ferry on Monday morning, nervous and
hopeful about embarking on their first-ever yoga retreat for
teen girls. It's Wednesday now, and all sixteen of them have
settled into the daily morning flow of the retreat: breakfast,
meditation, a yoga practice, journaling, and a circle discus-
sion. There have been secrets shared, tears shed, laughter,
and friendships made. I am always astounded by how quickly
connections are made at the retreat, but I know that's because
each day of a retreat can feel like a month. So much happens
in the waking hours of our days. We've already dug into so
much physical, mental and emotional work.

Her name is Sherice. She's seventeen years old. She's
cheerful but her eyes are full of sadness. For the first two
days she showed up to yoga wearing baggy hoodies. But
today she arrives in a sports bra and a newfound confidence.
She's different today. I can sense something has shifted.

Your yoga
teacher should
always ask for
consent before
touching you.

76

Everyone finds their yoga mat, places their journals down, splays their crystals and essential oils and other personal items decoratively around themselves. I can feel that the group is beginning to really vibe with yoga. We sit tall, close our eyes, and find our breath. Through slow inhales and exhales, everyone's breath is synced and sounds like a symphony of hope and release. I feel goosebumps rise on my flesh as I instruct the girls into movement. I can feel that this morning is a special morning.

Together we flow through the asana practice with ease. It is always mid-retreat where this fluidity forms, and it is as if we dance together in a choreographed rhythm. The music plays loud, the sweat drips, laughter and tears are ever present. Sherice has transformed in front of my eyes. She moves her body in a way that embodies a carefree freedom. Days ago, she could barely lift her arms over her head and now she reaches with vigor and grace.

As we near the end of class, we come onto our backs and set up for savasana. The Girlvana mentors, my team of camp counselors—slash—inspirational boss ladies—slash—big sisters, begin to move around the room. We have let everyone know that we will be coming around with essential oils to provide consensual touch to those who are open to being assisted into a deeper rest. (This is important. Make sure your yoga teacher always asks for consent before they touch you.)

I come to Sherice, who has her body laid out in a starfish shape with her arms above her head. In her previous savasanas she curled tightly into a fetal position, arms covering

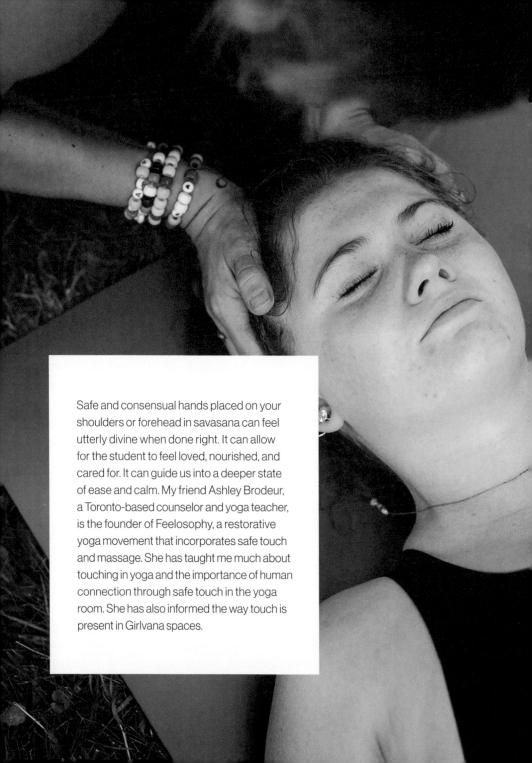

Safe and consensual hands placed on your shoulders or forehead in savasana can feel utterly divine when done right. It can allow for the student to feel loved, nourished, and cared for. It can guide us into a deeper state of ease and calm. My friend Ashley Brodeur, a Toronto-based counselor and yoga teacher, is the founder of Feelosophy, a restorative yoga movement that incorporates safe touch and massage. She has taught me much about touching in yoga and the importance of human connection through safe touch in the yoga room. She has also informed the way touch is present in Girlvana spaces.

and protecting her body. Today she has signaled that she is open to receiving touch and healing.

Before I come into place, my hands on her shoulders, I observe the openness she is expressing. She looks so peaceful and at home in her body. My eyes shift, and I begin to notice that the soft skin of her forearms abounds with tiny scars. I know these scars well. I have seen them on most of the teens I have taught throughout the years—tiny little slits made by razor blades. Cutting. A sharp slice that cuts through the darkness of the mind and a bright red bleed that makes you feel alive.

The scars have faded into tiny reminders of harder times. I kneel down and rub my hands together above her face to make my presence known. She inhales sharply as the smell of peppermint essential oil meets her nose. I place my hands instinctively on her forearms, directly on her scars, and she begins to sob. I stay there with the gentle pressure of my hands on her arms as she relaxes into the moment. I stay until she is calm again, my hands never leaving her arms. We share in a moment of connection and compassion. Eventually, I take her hands and squeeze them as if to say, *I am here. I am here for you.* So much can be communicated without a word.

I move back to the front of the room and close the class. I instruct everyone to make a circle once they have risen from the floor. We meditate and close the class with a deep breath, in and out. We open our eyes and begin to go around the circle, giving each girl a chance to express how she felt during the yoga practice. It can be a really powerful experience to share how we feel after yoga with the people we just practiced with. It is a time to express and feel seen.

Sherice goes first. She explains that no one has ever touched her scars. She says her parents can't stand them, her friends are embarrassed by them, and she feels broken when she sees them. She tells us that having her scars touched today was liberating. She cried deeply for who she was when she was cutting her flesh and she sees who she is now. The scars are a part of her story, but they do not define her anymore. Her worth is not defined by the marks on her body and instead of being ashamed by them, she feels powerful. Another teen says that the cracks are where the light gets in, and Sherice agrees knowingly. There was a reason she didn't wear her usual long-sleeved tee today, she says. She was ready to let us see all of who she is without shame.

It was time for Sherice to create a new narrative and through her willingness, she certainly did. Regardless of how she viewed her body or the ways she treated it in the past, she had come to embody kindness and acceptance for herself. This is our first yama, ahimsa, in action. Ahimsa teaches us to be non-harming in our thoughts, words, and actions towards ourselves and others (page 34). We can always begin again and use ahimsa as a guide on our journey of self.

79

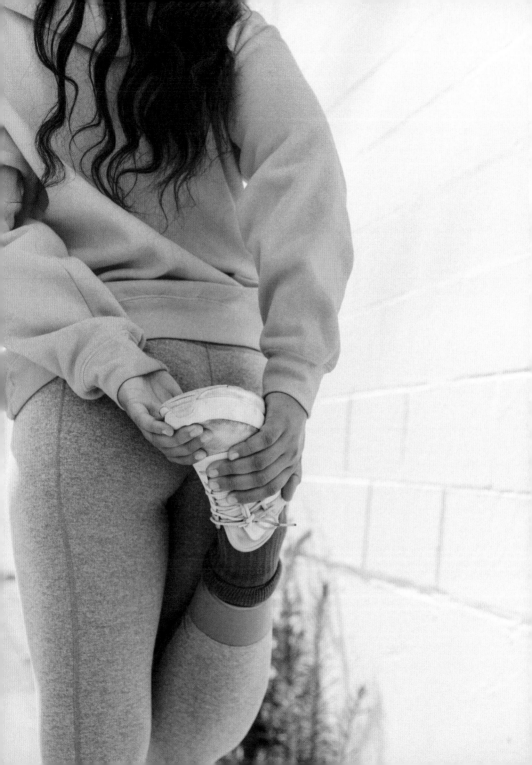

YOUR BODY

This chapter focuses on your body and aims to help you understand not only how to connect with it, but also how to befriend it. Ahimsa, non-harming, teaches us that being kind to ourselves is the first step in our journey to freedom. In this chapter we will look at why we feel bad about our bodies and how to begin to make peace with them.

I can't write a book for teen girls without addressing the relationship you have with your body. As I've said before, there are many messages that we receive as girls about what we should look like, how our value is wrapped up in physical perfection, and who our bodies are for. These messages can be confusing and damaging to our self-esteem and to our relationship with our bodies.

In Girlvana, we ask, *What does it mean to be truly in your body? What does it feel like to actually take up space in your physical form?* To me, yoga is all about living *in* the body. When we are in the body, we are in contact with the present moment. When we are in the present moment, we can access our wholeness.

Most of walk us around the world living only in the upstairs of our physical form. I often refer to this as the "attic" of our bodies. We live in our heads, overthinking, planning, dwelling, and overanalyzing, while the rest of the body becomes a receptacle of negative thoughts, unfelt emotions, shallow breaths, or weighty neglect.

Most of my teen life was spent in the attic, overthinking, always comparing myself to other people and housing toxic thoughts about myself and others. Yes, I was a dancer and was physically using my body, but that is all it was—using it. I had no concept of what it was like to take care of my body, let alone embody it. I had no clue that it was something to be honored or respected, so I wasn't able to demand respect or honor from someone else.

A YOUNG DANCER'S JOURNEY

From an early age I made my body the enemy. It never looked or felt the way I wanted it to, so I spent most of my time wishing it were different. I can't remember a time in my adolescent life when I enjoyed being in my body—for the most part I was always looking for ways to pick it apart. On especially bad days, I'd fantasize about crawling out of my skin, escaping reality, and getting as far away as I could from my own emotions. I felt trapped.

Growing up as a dancer meant that from a young age, I was constantly staring at myself in the mirror. Everything was about what my body could do and how it looked. Being a dancer trained me to become acutely aware of every inch of my body: the way my thighs touched, the deep curve in my lower spine, the length of my neck, the arch of my foot. My body was talked about at the ballet barre, or between my dance teachers and my parents, or on a ballet exam critique sheet. "Legs too muscular;" "Body is like a gymnast's;" "Torso is too long, legs too short, feet too flat"—my body was the reason I would never become a ballerina. I longed for the perfect "facility," as my dance teacher would call it. If only I were taller, leaner, and more flexible—maybe then I could have what I wanted. And what I wanted was to become a professional ballerina. I knew I had the heart, the passion, and even the talent, but I did not have the body. This detail was extremely clear to me, even as a tiny, innocent fifth grader.

When I was nine, I went to my very first ballet audition, for the National Ballet School of Canada. I remember being dressed in a navy-blue bodysuit, pink tights, and ballet slippers, and standing in a cold studio with sixty other girls my age. We were lined up perfectly in rows, tight buns and plastered smiles in place. We were told to take a quarter turn every sixteen bars of the piano music playing softly in the background. (To be clear, this was not a dance move; it was a way to see how our bodies were developing and what we looked like from all angles.) There was a stern yet poised woman at the front of the room simply watching and taking notes while our hopeful parents sat nervously behind her.

Soon after, we headed to the ballet barre to learn a few exercises. Excitedly, I thought this was my moment to shine; enough standing around, it was time to express and entertain. I had been working very hard for this moment and was eager for the chance to perform for others. But we executed just a few simple steps before moving back into a line.

We waited like statues with goose-bumped skin and numb toes, each of us anxiously hoping the number pinned to our chest would be called. If my number was called, I would be accepted into the National Ballet School of Canada, fulfilling my dream. If I didn't hear my number, I'd have to leave the studio immediately.

I did not hear my number that day. I was nine years old and I was devastated.

This would be my first memory of being judged solely on my body and what it looked like rather than for my talents or passions. That day was also when I decided that I was no longer good enough—a decision that sparked years of trying to prove my talents and worthiness.

THE STORIES WE BELIEVE

Even if you didn't grow up like I did, maybe you were also very aware of your body. Perhaps your mother made all of your "flaws" known, or maybe those "flaws" were the only thing you and your friends discussed. You see, the emphasis on the female body and what it should look like and how it should perform is connected to everything we do as women. From an early age, the message is clear: Your body is for the consumption of others, fair game for them to judge and have opinions about. From there, we decide our own worth. There are long-term effects of internalizing these messages as we grow up. In fact, my work with women aged thirty to

seventy (and even older) has proven to me that these messages never really leave us. They create a lasting imprint,
and if we aren't up for the task of undoing them, they can
cling to our souls forever.

What I have witnessed in so many of the girls I work with
is that we simply do not want to be held captive in our physical forms. We begin to view our bodies as objects, just like
society does, and then we end up disassociating from ourselves. Withdrawing from our bodies can feel like wanting to
escape. Where do we go and what do we do when we don't
want to feel the pain and discomfort of being in our bodies?

The answer to this could be getting lost in an internet
daze, undereating, overeating, purging, cutting (or other
forms of self-harm), unembodied sexual acts (for example,
doing it to please others), or getting high or blackout drunk.
Even if we hear from friends and family and believe to our
core that we are enough, the message saying otherwise is
persuasive, and it stays with us. And it doesn't help that
the media is constantly reaffirming this to keep us buying
makeup, fast fashion, "fit teas," and wellness programs. It's
really no wonder that on some level we internalize this
message and start to disassociate from our bodies, which,
in society's eyes, will never be perfect enough.

Whatever your story might be—whether your mom
forced you to step on a scale each morning; your ballet
teacher told you your thighs were too large; the boys at
your school made fun of your body for being too small, too
big, too curvy, or too whatever; or you never saw a body

that looked like yours being celebrated and accepted in mainstream media, we all have some sort of underlying narrative that says it is unsafe and uncomfortable to be in our bodies.

RUNNING TOWARDS YOURSELF

After a home invasion in my twenties in which I was very badly bear-maced by a male intruder, I felt even more disconnected from my body than I ever had before. My body was no longer a safe place to live. I felt victimized, taken

advantage of, and terrified to simply sit in my own skin that had been burned so badly. I have heard many girls and women describe this same experience of something being taken away from them physically, a feeling that their bodies are no longer theirs.

After the event, I began abusing my body with compulsive exercise and undereating to escape what I felt inside. I was terrified that if I slowed down and stopped running away, I might actually have to feel how scared and alone I was. On the outside I was the same bubbly girl going about her day, but on the inside I felt tortured, with no way out. I didn't know how to process what had happened to me. Did I deserve the attack? Was someone out to get me? Did I handle the situation properly? Should I have fought back? What could I have done differently? Was it my fault? These questions left me feeling empty and scared that I would never

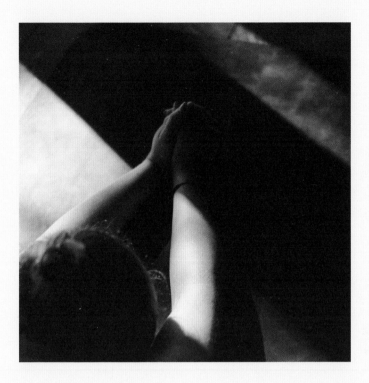

be the same. What if I could never fall asleep alone again, or what if I never felt safe again? I felt I had lost a sense of innocence, and I knew that the way I viewed the world had dramatically changed. I no longer felt like I belonged to myself.

After the attack I moved into a friend's in-law's home because I was too scared to be alone. I tried countless things to distract myself. I would spend the day exercising, sometimes for hours on end, then immediately need to be numbed by TV show after TV show. (Yes, Netflix, I am still watching.) If that didn't satisfy my desire to feel numb, I would

Who were
you before
the world
told you
who to be?

move on to drinking a bottle of wine by myself and eating multiple bowls of cereal. Each night, it was like I had the goal of drowning out every inch of fear through streaming services, booze, and Cheerios.

I would sleep with the lights on, with a fan going and a white noise app to fill the space. If I heard any movement at all through the night, I would wake up and my body would immediately freeze. I couldn't even get up and go to the bathroom during the night. The thought of moving my body even an inch was enough to paralyze me, so I would try to fall asleep in one position and force myself to stay there all night. I prayed for morning. As soon as the sun would rise, my dread would die down, but I would spend the rest of the day pretending like I wasn't scared and that everything was fine. After all, I felt like I *should* know better and that I *should* be over it by now. But the truth was that no amount of fitness, Netflix-watching, drinking, or binge eating was going to change how I felt inside.

My years of disordered eating and overexercising had taught me that the more I ran and hid from how I felt, the more isolated, scared, and lonely I would become. I knew this information, but I couldn't stop myself from those old patterns of coping.

I needed to ask for help. I sought out a therapist who specialized in post-traumatic stress disorder (PTSD), as well as a yoga teacher/mentor of mine. During this time, both my therapist and my mentor asked me to sit alone in my room, with no distractions, and simply breathe. Both of these wise women said that it was time for me to face my fear. I was instructed to recognize when the fear arose, when the loneliness arrived, and then the moment that I wanted to run. But I wasn't allowed to run. So I sat there, and when the terrifying ache arrived, I took a huge breath and met the fear. I breathed as deeply as I could while it threatened to overtake me.

The fear felt hot, hot like the bear mace. It felt suffocating, like the image of the man standing at the foot of my bed. The fear felt like a tsunami that was about to take me under. But I stayed with it, riding the feelings like waves, looking deep into the eyes of the loneliness. I would stay until the intensity subsided, which it always did. Sometimes it would take five minutes and sometimes a few hours, but I would sit and breathe and stay present with what was arising.

The work of staying with what was there versus immediately distracting myself to not feel the inevitable was the hardest thing I would do all day, but eventually it became easier and I felt braver, as well as a deep sense of pride when the huge waves of fear passed. Sometimes that meant letting myself come undone, sobbing, or doing whatever else I needed to do. But I did not run. I stayed.

THE ART OF FALLING APART

Before my break-in, I felt as if there was no space in my life to fall apart. I was terrified about the idea of unraveling.

Would I ever be able to piece myself together if I actually let it all go? I worried about losing friends or that people wouldn't understand. I was so used to being the strong one that if I fell apart around others they might see me as weak or incapable. So I took this time to fall apart in private. It was my little secret, a date I kept with myself so I could peel back my "I'm fine" mask, drop the heavy burden of what it felt like to be me, and just let myself release it all. Every night when I came home from work or class, I would eat my dinner and then sit alone with myself. Instead of being afraid to be alone, I began to enjoy it. It became peaceful. It felt powerful and healing.

I began to transition from seeing my loneliness as a bad thing to starting to become okay with being alone. I didn't have to label it as good or bad. Sitting with my fear became less scary, and slowly my need to numb out lessened and this okay-ness began to fortify me. It began to free me in a way I had never thought was possible. Over time, I no longer felt ashamed about my attack, nor did I blame myself. I began to open up to others about my PTSD, and through therapy and mentorship I was able to learn tools to work with it. The most profound step in all of this was truly my time spent alone, looking my fear in the eyes. In those moments of compelling, almighty darkness, I began to feel free and my body began to feel safe again.

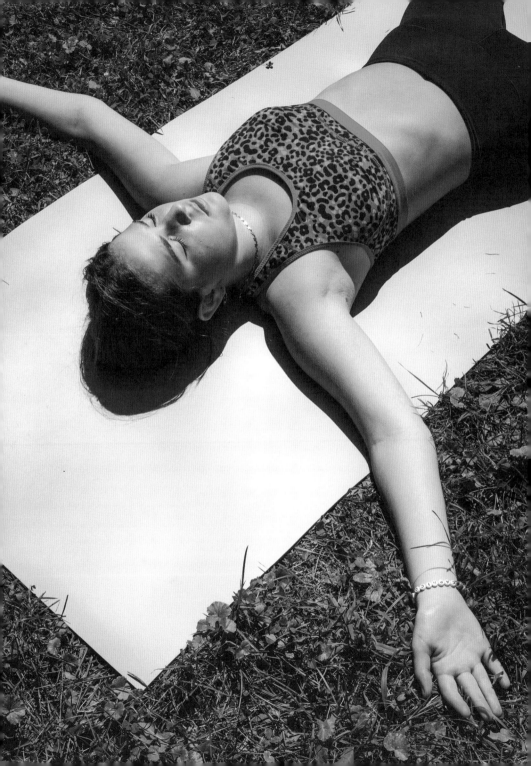

FEEL YOUR FEELINGS

I know that feeling safe in your body and with your emotions is possible for you too, because I know that the pain of running and hiding from what you feel is much greater than that of actually feeling it. The idea of *feeling your feelings* is a core message in Girlvana. You must give yourself the space and time to let yourself come undone, face the fear, and move through it. It took me time to come around to the idea that I was not okay. It is a slow process—maybe even one that's months long—and it can be incredibly intimidating, but it is powerful medicine.

You have heard this before, I am sure, but truly, the only way out is through. But if you ever feel like you simply cannot go on, having access to therapy or a school counselor is vital. Yoga has been there for me in countless ways, but sometimes we need a professional to assist us in this work and there is absolutely nothing wrong with that—in fact, I encourage it. There are plenty of online resources as well if you are curious about who or what type of professional you would like to talk to. I suggest starting with your school counselor or a trusted adult first.

TAKING UP SPACE

The way we can put this concept of being in our bodies into practice on a daily basis starts with breath. We can start by making our bodies, the place where we live, feel like a safe place.

Prior to finding yoga, I didn't necessarily notice that I was shrinking or hiding myself in my body. I equated sitting tall with selfishness instead of self-assuredness. As a teen, I never wanted to be seen as someone who was full of herself. The very thought of drawing my shoulders back made me feel like I was reveling in my body or showing off my boobs (or lack thereof). I didn't want the attention. Hunching forward and placing my hands around my waist were ways to hide. They were ways to be overlooked, and that somehow felt nobler than being some type of show-off with a straight spine. Why was I (along with so many other girls) afraid to stand up tall? Why does it feel strange or uncomfortable to take up space? Where did we learn to shrink?

The shift came when I began my yoga practice. Once I was more in my body, my perception of taking up space completely changed. I realized that to be full of oneself was a powerful thing! It was what we were all trying to achieve on that mat: to be able to fill our bodies with breath and claim the bodies that belonged to us was liberating.

Through my practice I was able to identify what caused me to shrink and when. I noticed moments when I didn't know how to stand tall, because doing so made me feel self-conscious. Maybe I didn't think I deserved to be there, or maybe I thought the other yoga students would judge me if I lifted my head and puffed my chest proudly. But, slowly, yoga helped me to see that when negative thoughts

93

took over my mind, my movements or poses would become lifeless, or I would just give up and crawl back into child's pose. It took me some time to learn how to stand strong and how to show up for challenging moments. I learned that I deserve to breathe and move big, not just on my mat but in the world.

STAND TALL

Something I've noticed as a yoga instructor is that when a girl is new to yoga her movement is often smaller, more timid, and a bit uncertain. Something as simple as standing in *tadasana* (mountain pose, which is two feet on the ground, arms beside the body, eyes forward) can feel silly, uncomfortable, or even shameful.

When we practice standing tall and taking up space on our yoga mats, it can translate off the mat and into our "regular" lives as well: our confidence rises and a sense of self develops. We begin to learn that the body is a powerful place to step into and embody. So, it is our time to take up space in this world. To practice, give this simple and mighty pose a try.

TADASANA (MOUNTAIN POSE)

A Practice in Taking Up Space

1. Stand with your feet hip-width apart.

2. Let your arms relax at your sides.

3. Draw your shoulder blades together so your chest is open and proud.

4. Lift your chin up.

5. Set your gaze forward.

6. Breathe here for five breaths, feeling your strength and inner presence.

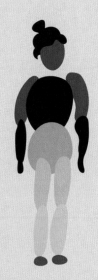

Mountain pose

95

TRUE POWER

When our thoughts are overriding our presence, our breath tends to be short and unconscious. This shallow breathing means we are sending less oxygen to our brain and that we aren't functioning at our optimum level. When we are in the attic of our minds, our bodies have less power and presence. From an outsider's view, we might be seen as susceptible prey.

When we are "in the body," all senses are sharper. When we stand taller, we appear more confident, and we command presence and elicit self-assuredness. And this is the kind of skill that emboldens others to find their own innate strength. This is not the kind of power that takes from others. What we are cultivating through embodiment is the *true power*, the kind that doesn't hurt, steal, or lie. It lifts, inspires, and strengthens everything and everyone around it.

I want you to start putting this into practice. Take. Up. Space. Start with big breaths that move you out of your attic and into the home that is your body. Then start to practice sitting, walking, and standing with purpose wherever you are, be it in the cafeteria, on the bus, or at the dinner table with your family. Move with bigness and intention. Stretch your arms high and wide. Walk with pride. Lift your chin. Look people in the eye. It can help to check in with what parts of your body are making contact with your chair, the floor, or your clothing. Claim your space in this world; it is your time. You are allowed to be here. When you do this, you give permission to other women to do the same.

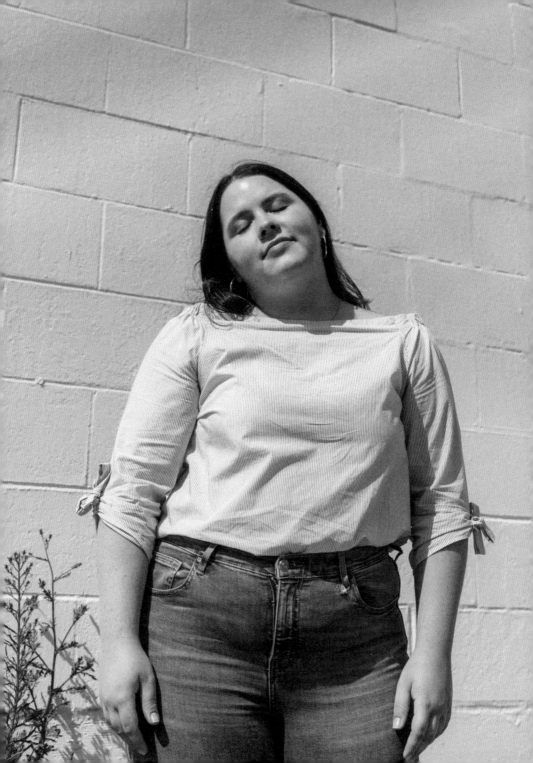

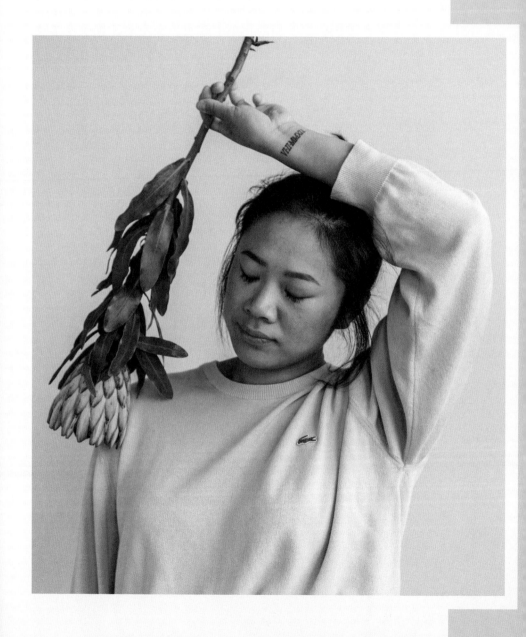

BREATH RETENTION

Once we begin to understand how to breathe with awareness by elongating our inhales and exhales, we can begin to explore a greater range of lung capacity. This breathing exercise gets us to really take up space in our bodies by testing the space we have to take in breath, hold it, and then release it fully. Notice how each time you hold your breath, you are able to make a bit more space inside of yourself. This breath is also known as box breathing and can be a beautiful compliment or addition to any of your meditations.

1. Inhale through the nose for four counts.

2. Hold the breath in for four counts.

3. Exhale through the nose or mouth for four counts.

4. Hold the breath out for four counts.

5. Repeat for a minimum of ten complete breath cycles.

99

When we make space within, we can feel more relaxed and also alert. Use this breathing exercise whenever you feel like you need more room for yourself to exist.

NAVIGATING OUR PERIODS

The body holds an incredible amount of wisdom and intelligence. When we are able to tune in, listen, and be *in* our bodies, the more we can interpret what our bodies are trying to tell us. In turn, we can make better decisions and start to really take care of ourselves.

Part of taking care of our bodies is to honor what they naturally go through for those whose body produces a menstrual cycle. One of the most intelligent things our bodies can do is have a period. Learning about our cycles can help us better understand our emotions and our mental health. Yet the narrative around periods is that they are something to hide, that they make us crazy, and that we should be disgusted and ashamed by them. So, by learning about our cycles, we take back the power in our bodies and reclaim what society has deemed taboo, unclean, or a curse.

How did something so natural become so embarrassing?
When I first got my period, no one was really there to talk to me about what I was feeling or what it meant. I was at a dance recital when I noticed the brownish stain on my ballet tights. I panicked and quickly jammed a Tampax "teen" tampon inside me and kept going. A few days later I wrote my mom a letter and told her to absolutely never bring my period up to me, ever. I also wrote, *Whatever you do, do NOT tell Dad!* Even though getting my period was something I had been anticipating and sort of wanted, I felt so humiliated and sad.

I was also terrified that a massive gush of blood was going to burst through me at any given moment, as I walked down the hall at school. And with my period came terrible cramps and skin breakouts that made me feel uncomfortable, ugly, and completely unmotivated.

Soon after, when I was fourteen, I was put on birth control to control the cramps and to clear my skin. The pill was sold to me as the cure-all for everything I was experiencing as a teen. As it turned out, dancers at my studio used the pill back to back to make sure that we didn't get our periods during dance competitions and ballet exams. In the beginning it seemed like a magic fix. But the subject still felt so taboo at the time that I never really discussed it with my mom. It was a quick solution and made life seemingly easier, so I truly never thought that there could be any repercussions.

The truth was that at such a young age I was already being taught that my period was something to deny and get rid of. It was something my friends and I were embarrassed about, hiding tampons up our sleeves before running to the bathroom at school. It was something we thought of as a curse, something to despise and blame as the source of our mood swings, weight gain, acne, and low productivity.

It wasn't until my mid-twenties that I embarked on a quest to make peace with my period. I was getting deeper into yoga and was starting to honor my body and nourish my spirit, but my disordered eating had stopped my cycle entirely for over a year. I felt like I was missing a huge part of myself. It was only then that I finally recognized that having a period was a sign of good health and provided a balance to my body, something that I was suddenly yearning for.

Getting my period back was a journey of looking deeply at my battles with my body. Finally, through a healthier relationship with food and exercise, my period returned, and I vowed to honor it and keep my body a welcoming place. The more I respected my time of the month, the more connected and powerful I felt.

It was like an act of rebellion to love my period, even in my friend group. I hadn't ever met anyone who embraced their period. It seemed like hating and complaining about your period was something all women did. I began reading anything I could find about the magic of periods and the divine energy within us all. I began to sync my cycle with the moon, and I intuitively started to create ritual and ceremony around the different times of my cycle each month. Through lots of research, I landed with a deeper understanding of the seasons we go through each month as menstruating humans. I say menstruating *humans* because it isn't just a cisgender (born into a body you identify with) female thing to bleed each month. It is important to include trans and nonbinary people within this conversation, too.

SEASONS OF OUR CYCLES

Once my period came back, I became obsessed with learning more and more about it. One of the most influential teachers in this work is my friend Carly Rae Beaudry. She does a lot of work in the area of women's reproductive health, and she really shifted the way I view and take care of my body, especially my menstrual cycle.

The information below has come from many years of research, Carly's guidance and affirmation, and my own experience. You can use this to develop a new relationship with your own period.

Think of each cycle of your period as a year with different seasons. Just like "real" seasons, your body will need different things based on the season you're in.

103

Winter

This season marks the first day of your cycle—the first day you bleed.

This season can last between one and eight days.

The key themes during this time are *hibernate* and *rest*.

This is time to give to *yourself* and not to others.

Ask yourself, *What can I let go of? What pattern, habit, or negative thought needs to die or end during this cycle?*

Tips for Optimizing This Season
+ Keep yourself warm, especially your feet!
+ It's okay to be less social, so cancel plans if you feel like you need to. Practice the mantra *I am honoring myself right now and saying no to plans.*
+ Take the chance to spend time alone.
+ Use this time to explore your creativity: write, read, and journal.
+ Use organic cotton period products, a menstrual cup, and/or period underwear. They're better for you and the environment.
+ Make friends with your body. See your period as an inner ceremony of release and renewal. Think of the blood as a release of toxic energy and whatever else feels stagnant, or stuck, in you.

Spring

This season, also known as the follicular phase, typically begins on day seven of your cycle and lasts until day thirteen.

The key themes during this time are *rebirth* and *fresh start.*

You will likely feel energetic and focused during this time, thanks to the estrogen in your body rising, so it's a great time to get things done.

Tips for Optimizing This Season
+ Use this time to plan and be productive. You'll feel more energetic, so finish stuff like your homework, finances, and big projects that require lots of focus.
+ Work out, move your body—this is the time to move, while your body has the most energy.

Summer

This season usually lasts from day fourteen of your cycle until day twenty-one. During this time, ovulation occurs.

The key themes during this time are *self-expression* and *being social*, so it's a great time to ask for what you want. Be bold!

This is also a good time to nurture others and find ways to be of service.

Tips for Optimizing This Season
+ This is the most fertile time in your cycle, which means that you have the highest chance of

becoming pregnant, so use protection or avoid
having sex at this time.

• This is a good time to go for a job interview, or
do something you've been afraid of doing . . . ask
someone on a date, maybe?

• This is a great time to connect with your friends
and to hold space for them. Think of ways you can
help them and others.

Fall

This cycle typically begins on day twenty-two of
your cycle and ends on day twenty-nine. This phase
is known as the luteal phase.

The key theme for this season is *winding down.*

This is the time in your cycle when PMS can
occur, and you may notice that you are more
irritable or tired.

Tips for Optimizing This Season

• This is the time to slow things down. Start to limit
your social calendar, be less physically active, and
increase your self-care practices. Your hormones
are dipping, and it's important to honor that.

- This is a good time to assert boundaries and begin looking inward. Don't compare yourself to your spring or winter self.
- Find ways to express your creativity. Slowing down and listening can lead to lots of inspiration.

Once I began to recognize these seasons within myself, I was able to give myself what I needed during specific weeks of my cycle. I learned that slowing down during the fall and winter seasons of my cycle allowed for more energy during the spring and summer seasons. I also found that I had the energy and space to better support those around me. Before, during my fall and winter weeks, I would typically become very stressed, depressed, and overwhelmed; now I feel more creative, intuitive, and nurturing. I also began to notice when my self-esteem and mental health would plummet in relation to my cycle, so I could catch myself, pump the brakes, and take the rest I needed to find harmony.

I used to believe that taking that time was lazy and unproductive, and deep down I felt that I didn't deserve it. But there is nothing lazy about a female, or any human, taking care of themselves. In fact, space and time to reflect and recharge is necessary. Do not feel guilty for needing time alone or saying no to others. Honoring your seasons will serve you well. The more you can learn about your body, the more you can love the intelligent and miraculous thing that it is.

Taking up space and being in
our bodies is a radical act. It is
a political act, and it can most
definitely disrupt industries and
change the world. Embodying
yourself is a necessary action
in knowing yourself.

108

This meditation is designed to connect
you with the first yama: ahimsa, or nonviolence (page 34). When I am feeling
off, the first question I ask myself is,
Am I being kind to myself? This meditation
is designed to reactivate kindness within
ourselves and set us back on the path of
being more compassionate humans.

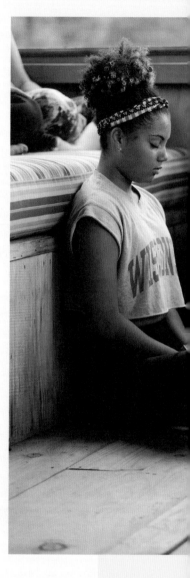

AHIMSA MEDITATION

1. Make yourself comfortable by sitting
   or lying down.

2. Close your eyes and begin to breathe
   deeply.

3. Take a moment to ask yourself, *How
   have I been treating myself lately?* Try not
   to judge whatever comes up in response;
   just listen.

4. As you continue to breathe, forgive
   yourself for anything you have said
   internally to beat yourself up or anything
   you have said that has caused harm to
   you or others.

5. As you inhale, breathe in the words
   I forgive you.

6. As you exhale, breathe out the words
   I am forgiven.

7. Repeat ten times.

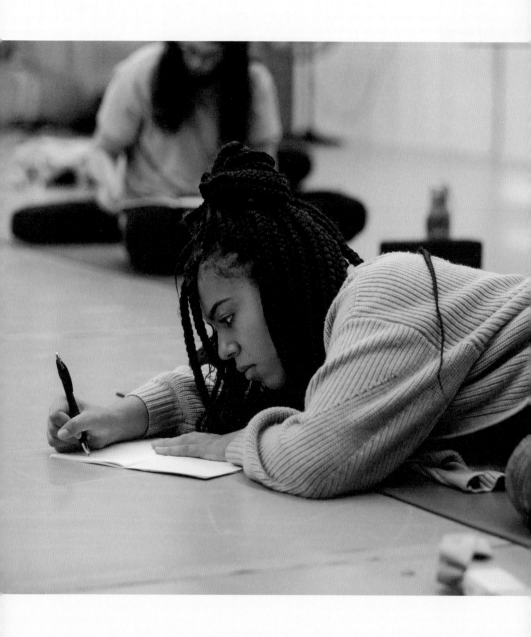

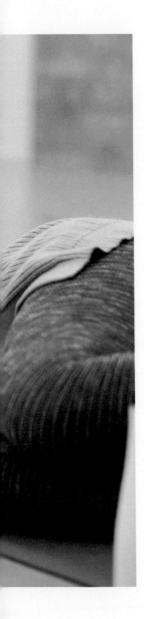

JOURNAL

This is a writing activity that I have used in retreats for both teens and women for the last decade: a letter to your body. I find it's a really powerful way to check in on your relationship to your body, and to bring ahimsa to life through your words. All that is needed is an honest heart and time to breathe.

As you write, you may find that what pours from you is a thank you, a forgiveness, a celebration of all that your body has been through. Sometimes this exercise brings up past hurt or anger and that is okay too. Allow what needs to move, to move through you.

I'm sharing a letter that Mici, a brilliant teen from Vancouver, British Columbia, wrote when she was thirteen and at her first Girl-vana retreat. To this day, it remains one of my favorite "Dear Body" letters of all time.

III

Dear Body,

I'm sorry for treating you like a rundown motel, like something I feel gross even touching. But you are more than a room I sleep only one night in. You are my home, a place of safety, sanctuary, and pure gratitude. But still, I forget.

I'm sorry I was convinced I deserved no home when you were there all along. Me neglecting you was only a product of me being neglected. And the society that taught me I was only checked into my body for a weekend getaway is the same society that sleeps homeless each night.

Please hear my cries when I say I love you now. When I say you are my home in a beautiful neighborhood with a big backyard and a kitchen made for nourishment.

I promise I will never leave home again.

YOUR TURN.

the power of
your mind

"Girlvana transformed
ideas like staying true
to myself and trusting
my gut from cliché
quotes into words I live
by. Girlvana helped me
meet my most true and
authentic self."

—Amelie, 15,
ST. STEPHEN, NEW BRUNSWICK

03

PRIYA

Her name is Priya and she is seventeen. She is a thoughtful, insightful, and wildly intelligent young woman. She is the recipient of a full scholarship to attend the Girlvana summer retreat after writing a beautiful and poignant application rooted in her quest for spirituality and gender equality and her desire to learn more about yoga and feminism. I was so excited to meet this clever girl and get to know her better.

We get girls from all walks of life at the retreat, but the truth is, many of them are forced by their parents, counselors, or teachers to attend. But some, like Priya, actually *want* to come. In fact, Priya's family was the opposite of encouraging when it came to her being here. It is not in the culture of her family to discuss your problems with other people, let alone strangers. In their eyes, it's impolite or even humiliating to have your daughter share her innermost feelings with a group. Young girls have no business being messy, emotional, or all "Kumbaya"-like. But Priya wants to be here and has assured her parents that this is what she wants, that it is healthy to share with and be around like-minded teens. She arrives at the retreat eager and ready.

Each morning Priya sets up her yoga mat in the front row, lays out her journal and pen in a neat and tidy way, and sits patiently waiting for the class to begin. She strikes me as someone who doesn't want to waste a single opportunity. She is kind and patient with the other girls, but her presence expresses that she is a sponge and she is here to learn.

We begin to dive into the topic at hand: the second of the yamas, satya, which means "truth." I start by asking the group, "Are all the thoughts in our head true?" At first no one answers. It is a complex question.

Priya raises her hand slowly and asks, "Is it the ego that is thinking?" I ask her to expand on that. She tells us about a book that she read and how it described the ego as a voice in everyone's head that can be hurtful. "For example," she continues, "I can hear this voice sometimes telling me I am not good enough, that I will never be good enough, and that I don't matter. But then when we do yoga or meditate, that voice gets quieter and I feel better, happier." I nod encouragingly as she goes on. "This voice is always negative! Do this, do that, why did you say that? It is never-ending. I feel like I am constantly battling it." Priya's voice is getting louder and her body language more animated. I can tell she has been wanting to have this conversation and ask these questions for a while now, but like most young people, she probably doesn't have anyone to talk about this with.

"I hear all of this *just be positive* kind of stuff, but how? How do we actually stop thinking all of these negative thoughts? How do we stop it?" The whole class nods in agreement, but I can feel a bit of shock coming from them. *Are we really talking about the voice in our heads? Other people hear that, too?* All of a sudden, this yoga camp has become a touch more interesting for everyone. It feels as though this conversation is revealing one of life's greatest yet least discussed mysteries.

"I hear my thoughts, that voice, go on and on and on," Priya is saying, "and then in yoga or when we meditate, it calms down and I hear another voice . . . a kinder one, maybe? Who or what is that?" She is looking more inquisitive than ever.

I pause and let everyone digest these questions. I know that some of them must be feeling a little overwhelmed and paying extra attention to this voice inside their heads now. I tell them that the first step is awareness. Can we become aware of this voice? Can we listen to what it has to say? The group takes a moment to listen.

Then I ask, "What does the voice in your head tell you?" The answers begin to popcorn into the space:

I am worthless.
I am dumb.
I am ugly.
I am fat.

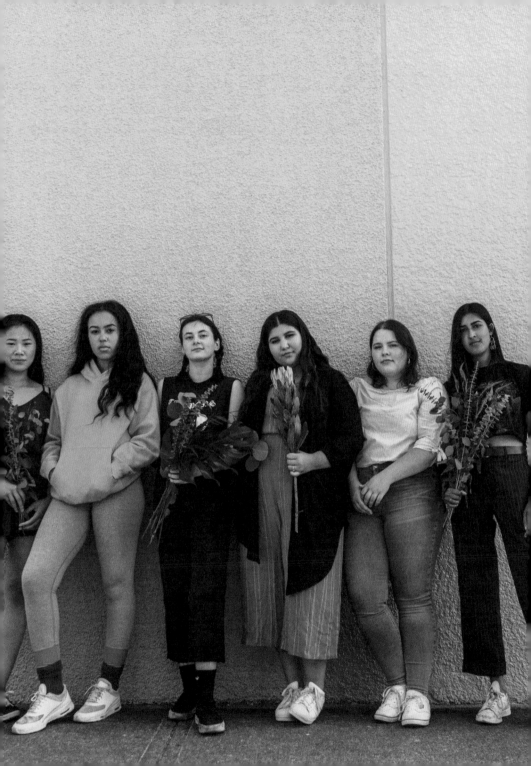

Am I doing this right?
Why even try?
No one likes me.
She is prettier than me.
I will never be good enough.
I will never be happy.
Do they like me?
I will always be depressed.
I will be anxious forever.
Do I look stupid?
Will I sound stupid?

The list goes on and on, and a buzzy excitement fills the room, the kind that is created when we have a shared experience. All of a sudden, these young women feel as though they belong. They feel relieved.

"Even if I get an A on a test, I still don't feel good enough."

"Yeah, for me, when something great happens, I worry that I don't deserve it."

"Same! Like I don't really deserve to be happy."

"Or if I am happy, people will think I am being selfish . . ."

"I always worry that if I am actually being myself, people won't accept me."

"Exactly, I feel like I have to always watch what I say to make sure I am fitting in—"

"—And then I beat myself up for trying to fit in! Or trying to stand out! Or doing anything!"

Priya looks at me earnestly and asks, "So how do we make it stop?"

Great question!

BECOMING AWARE OF OUR THOUGHTS

When I was fifteen, I was at a sleepover with friends (like we did each weekend). I remember being in the bathroom washing my hands and looking in the mirror. I was acutely aware that the reflection staring back at me was my body, but I felt for the first time that I didn't recognize myself. I remember meeting my own gaze and feeling foreign to myself. I could hear my thoughts loudly, I could see my body, but I couldn't make sense of the difference. Was I my body? Was I my mind? Who was I? Who was thinking?

The questions terrified me. I had never been aware of my thoughts before; I just sort of thought them. I had never looked in the mirror and really looked beyond what I had deemed ugly, fat, and not good enough. It was like I woke up in someone else's body, with someone else's thoughts.

Later that night, as we were curled up on the floor in sleeping bags in my friend's living room, I cautiously asked, "Have you ever looked in the mirror and not recognized yourself?"

One of my friends burst out laughing. "What are you talking about?"

"You know," I began, "when you stare at yourself in the mirror but you don't really know who you are. Like you are thinking thoughts but they are really loud and they don't feel like your own?" My friends continued to laugh, cracking jokes like I was being abducted by aliens. *Maybe I sounded absolutely insane,* I thought. So I pretended I was joking and was just trying to make them laugh.

I didn't really sleep that night. I had so many unanswered questions about my thoughts and why they felt so loud, and why my body felt foreign to me. The only thing that I knew for certain was that sharing those questions with other people was no longer an option. So I buried them and tried to avoid looking at or hearing myself like that again.

It wasn't until my first yoga teacher training course years later, when I was twenty-one years old and my teacher, Shakti Mhi, asked us the question that I had asked myself when I was fifteen—"Who is thinking?"—that it felt like I was finally getting an answer to this secret question I had kept hidden for so long.

So to answer my fifteen-year-old self and sweet Priya's question, I have created a step-by-step process to identify our thoughts, shine a light on the ego, and ultimately release the thoughts that are causing us harm. When we are able to do this, we can rest easier in our own bodies and minds.

RECOGNIZE, ASK, RELEASE

Ahimsa means "non-harming," and *satya* means "truth."

Recognize: First, we must become aware of our thoughts. We must consciously recognize that we are thinking in order to break the trance-like state of unconsciousness. Ask yourself, *What am I thinking?* Sometimes it is helpful to make a list or speak it out loud.

Ask: Once you are aware of your thoughts, ask, *Is that true?* and let your heart answer. When we inquire about truth, we are bringing our satya practice to life.

Release: Let go of the thoughts that are harmful to your well-being. This is how ahimsa is connected to satya. When you release the negative self-talk, you can access peacefulness and liberation.

124

It is actually possible to choose differently for yourself once you become aware of your thoughts. Your awareness catches your thoughts in the act and says, *Hey, is that really true?* Then you get to decide if those thoughts are harming you or helping you. When we illuminate our thoughts like this, they become less powerful. It's like looking under the bed for the bogeyman. When we turn the light on and check under the bed, the bogeyman isn't actually there. This is the power of satya. It helps us dive beyond the surface and connect to what is real.

We are the presence that is beyond the mind and body.

The Ego: The Small Self

Let's make an important distinction here. This voice inside your head, the one that is always thinking, is called the ego. The ego loves to create separation and makes us feel unworthy or othered by comparison. Every time we are able to become aware of our thoughts, the ego weakens. I like to call the ego my small self, because when I listen to the ego, I shrink. The ego is obsessively preoccupied with identifying with and attaching itself to things: what we look like, who we know, what we have. The ego feeds off of comparing itself with others. When we are not paying attention to our thoughts, it is the ego who is running the show.

Awareness: The Higher Self

When we bring consciousness to our thoughts, we can identify the ego. We can call this action presence, awareness, observance, or our higher Self. The higher Self can watch the ego and dissolve its power over us. The quickest way for me to get to that point is to ask myself, *Is that true?* I remind my students all the time that the ego is a liar and to not always believe everything you think. When we can give voice to the ego, we can then choose to believe it or not. Believing the ego keeps us trapped. Becoming aware of the ego frees us.

OH, HEY EGO!

It is important for me to point out that "Recognize, Ask, Release" is a forever practice. I find myself doing this multiple times a day. If I am feeling bad about myself and in a funk, it takes me a moment to remember and to catch myself: *Oh right, what is the thought I am thinking right now?* Once I identify the negative talk, comparison, judgment, overanalyzing, or doubt that is going on, I will say, *Oh, hey ego!* Even just acknowledging the ego feels like a great relief. Then, I dig a little deeper by asking, *Is the thought I am having true?* More times than not, it is the same self-deprecating noise that is harming me. I then ask myself, *Can I let this go?* Sometimes I can, but if not, I stay present by focusing on my breath and waiting for the storm to pass.

QUIET MIND

You see, it is not necessarily about replacing each negative thought with a positive one—that can feel fake or forced, like placing a Band-Aid over a wound that is still bleeding and pretending everything is fine. Sometimes it is simply about quieting the mind and bringing awareness to the ego. We don't have to be perky and positive to feel better, but we do have to be brave. Brave enough to face the ego and bring light to the dark thoughts and choose to release them in order to keep our minds free and safe from harm.

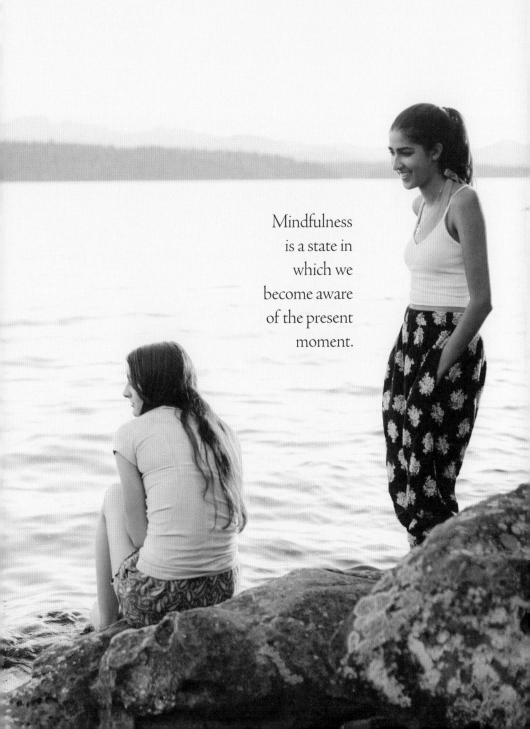

Mindfulness is a state in which we become aware of the present moment.

WHAT IS MINDFULNESS?

Our minds
are incredibly
powerful.
What we think
dictates our
beliefs and our
actions.

128

These days, *mindfulness* is a major buzzword. Let's unpack what it truly means to be mindful. Mindfulness is a mental state in which we become aware of the present moment. The present moment is defined as the here and now. It is not the past and it is not the future. It is in this very moment and it is in this very breath. It is where we can be aware of our thoughts, our feelings, and our bodies—but we are not controlled or defined by our thoughts.

Remember that our goal with yoga and meditation is not to stop our thinking minds entirely; rather, our intention is to become aware of them and not let them completely hijack us or derail us out of the present moment.

Pema Chödrön, a beloved Buddhist teacher, author, and nun, has said, "You are the sky, everything else is just the weather." If we can pull back and watch our thoughts and emotions like a passing storm, we can stay grounded and centered in who we are, and our thoughts and feelings will have less of a hold over us. Remember that *no thought is forever and no feeling is forever.*

WHAT IS ANXIETY?

Anxiety is the body's response to stress. Many describe anxiety as an unruly feeling living in their chest or belly. To me, it is this incessant panicky feeling that makes it hard to focus on what I'm doing and prevents me from living my life fully. Anxiety can hold us back from so much, from getting menial tasks done, to having the confidence to leave the house, to being able to have a social life. Anxiety can block us from feeling joy and peace.

One of the most anxiety-inducing things we do is listen to our negative thoughts and believe that they are real. Or we try to ignore them and push them down. Neither of these options gives us release from the grip of the ego. The only way we can come back to a sense of calm and peace is to address the fact that these thoughts exist. And instead of running from them—as dark, mean, or harsh as they are—we need to look at them dead-on. So I will often say to myself, *Okay, I am afraid. I feel scared,* and instead of letting the thoughts take me over, I just stay with the feeling. It's important to name the thought or feeling you're experiencing. By saying *I am scared,* you are taking away some of the power that the feeling has over you. When you can elaborate (for example, *I feel scared because* . . .), it creates space for you to breathe and become less attached to and consumed by what is going on.

The mind can be very tricky terrain to navigate. It can be filled with lots of irrational thoughts that are hard to make sense of, and it's the place where the ego can take us down some deep spirals of shame, doubt, worthlessness, and comparison (the ego *loves* to compare). It is important to understand that the ego wants to live anywhere *but* the present moment.

129

You are the sky— everything else is just the weather.

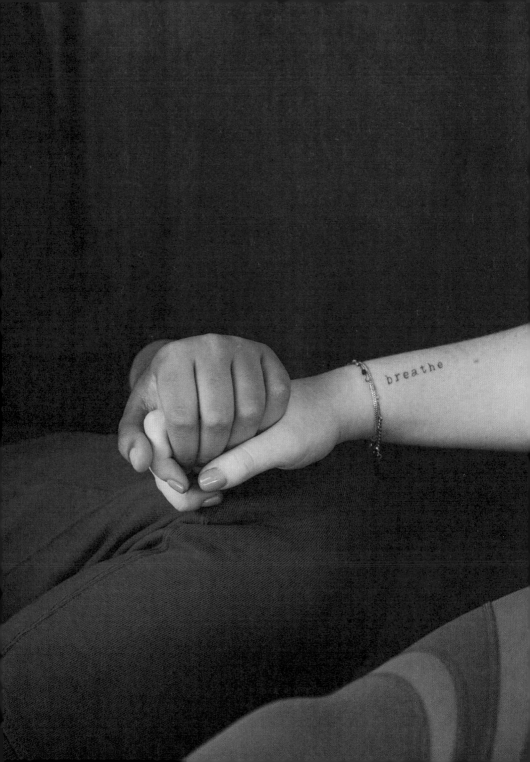

TIPS FOR ANXIETY

1. When you begin to feel anxious, it is best to identify it immediately, instead of trying to pretend you're fine. When we leave it unaddressed, it will build. The ego thrives in that unconscious place. Start by saying, *I feel anxious.*

2. Begin to deepen your breath and give those anxious feelings more space. As someone who has suffered many asthma and panic attacks, I find focusing on slowing down my breath is the number one tool I have to start calming myself down. Breathing slowly to regulate your nervous system will help you begin to feel calmer.

3. Once you identify the anxiety and get a handle on a deeper breath, ask yourself, *What do I need right now?* This question gives us options. Often when we are anxious, we feel trapped. When we ask this simple question, it allows us to feel acknowledged and cared for.

4. Make a choice. Do you need to lie down and rest, do you want to do something productive, do you need to go for a walk? What can you give yourself in this moment?

Remember that you are your own best friend. You can take care of yourself.

Acknowledge, breathe, and choose. Repeat as needed.

131

WHAT IS DEPRESSION?

Depression is classified as a mood disorder that can result in feelings of ongoing sadness. I think everyone at some point in their life can relate to the feelings associated with both anxiety and depression. Yoga has been proven to support those who suffer from depression and anxiety through its regulation of stress using breath, movement, and focus.

Throughout my life I have battled off and on with depression, and while my depression has in no way been completely "cured" by yoga, my yoga practice and breathing exercises have helped a great deal. And over the years I've seen how they've helped countless teens whom I've worked with. But I also know that when we are depressed, often the simplest task, like getting out of bed or doing a breathing exercise, can feel incredibly overwhelming.

TIPS FOR DEPRESSION

What helps me through those depressive spells is this strategy:

+ Commit to one small task at a time. Get out of bed and brush your teeth and take a shower. I find that cleaning myself up is a really good start.

+ Once I complete those small tasks, I try and focus on the next simple task, like making the bed. If I can make the bed amidst my own internal chaos or sadness, I feel as though I have accomplished something big. Even if the rest of the day goes to hell, I have a space that is tidy that I can come back to. (It might sound silly to you, or like your mom is ghostwriting this book right now, but making the bed is honestly one of my greatest tools to begin to break me out of a hard time. A simple act of caring for yourself can reorient you. Instead of becoming overwhelmed by every single thing you have to do, take it one task at a time and reevaluate from there.)

133

+ Beyond focusing on one task at a time, keeping up with a regular movement and breath practice is the best preventative action we can take. I've noticed my mental health often slips the most when I have been neglecting yoga.

+ A powerful breathing exercise I have in my toolkit is the breath of fire. This exercise has, time and time again, helped me to move stagnant and helpless energy from my body. When you oxygenate yourself, you have more energy, and when you have energy, you can get up and start to take care of yourself again.

BREATH OF FIRE

The Sanskrit name for the breath of fire is *kapalabhati*, which translates into "shining skull breath." This *pranayama* (breathing exercise) heats the body from the inside out, making you feel alive, awake, and full of energy. I do this breath almost every morning to kick-start my day. It wakes me up from feeling sluggish, and it helps calm my nervous system and relax any anxieties I may have. Try it—it's an instant mood elevator, especially if you are feeling low.

1. Sit tall, cross-legged or kneeling.

2. Make a cup shape with each hand and have your palms face the ceiling.

3. Keeping this cup shape, reach your arms overhead.

4. Inhale through your nose, and immediately sharply exhale from your nose. As you exhale, feel your belly button snap back toward your spine.

5. Repeat, focusing only on your exhale. Don't worry; the inhale will come naturally.

6. Start with 50 exhales and work your way up to 200.

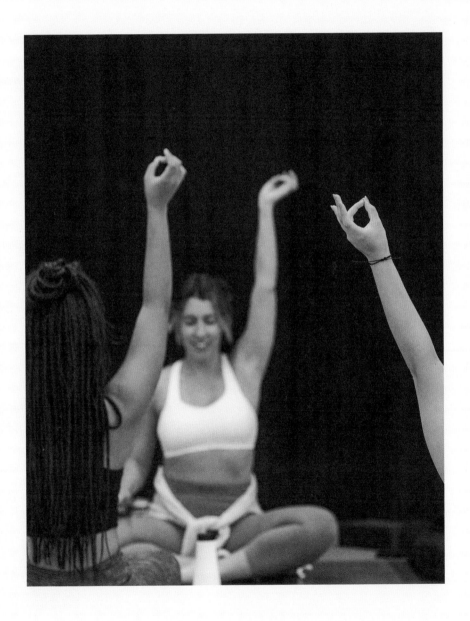

FINDING THE TRUTH

For me, yoga is the practice of finding my
own truth. As a teen, I was more focused
on being cool or perfect than I was inter-
ested in what I wanted and felt. My own
truth was never something that I knew
how to explore.

Through the practice of satya, we are
shown ways to see that not everything we
think is true. In our quest to live a more
peaceful and joyful life, it is essential to
discern what we think. Being in the constant practice of *Is that true?* can help us
reorient ourselves away from the false
thoughts spinning out of control in our
minds. We must be able to identify when
the ego is pulling us down.

I had a student, Megan, who named her
ego Sheryl. Every time Megan felt like
she was beating herself up, she would say,
"Stop it, Sheryl!" By naming her ego, she
was able to stop it in its tracks when
things were getting harmful in her mind.

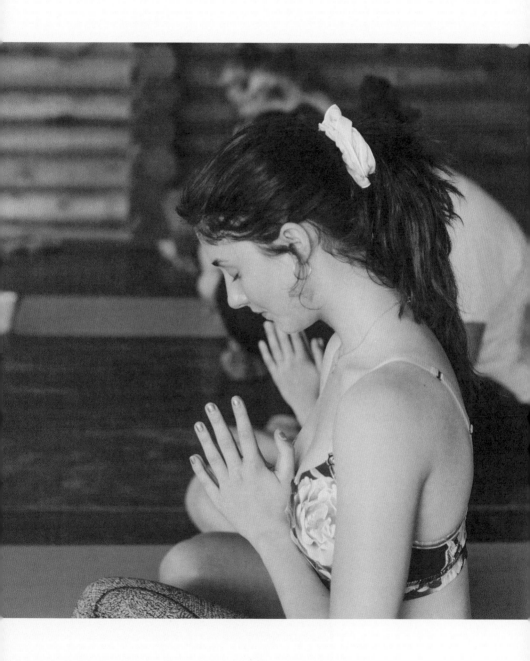

SATYA MEDITATION

This is a meditation designed to help you let go of the ego and to reconnect you to your truth. Use this when you are feeling down about yourself or are feeling beat up by your own thoughts.

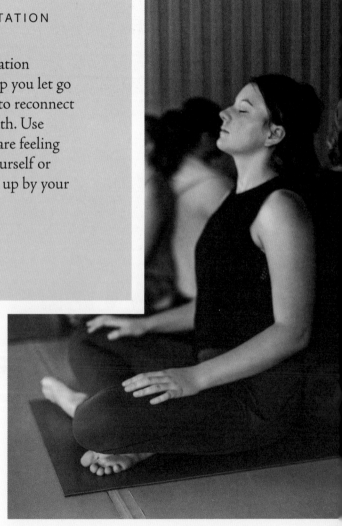

1. Find a comfortable place to sit or lie down and close your eyes.

2. Notice where you feel your breath. Do you feel it in your chest? Can you sense that the breath is shallow or quick?

3. Begin to slow your breath down to long inhales and exhales. I like to aim for a four-beat inhale and a four-beat exhale.

4. Start to simply "watch" your thoughts. Notice what it is that you're thinking. Imagine that your thoughts are being projected in front of you, like a movie. You are the watcher, the one who is observing these thoughts.

5. If you get carried away with your thoughts, come back to your breath. Let it guide you back to the present moment.

6. Ask yourself whether the thoughts you are thinking are true, and let your highest Self answer for you.

7. As you exhale, release the ego's thoughts.

8. Notice if the mind can take a bit of a break from thinking. Sense if there is a place inside your mind that is free of thought.

9. Start with practicing this for three minutes and work your way up to ten minutes.

A PRACTICE IN PRESENCE

During your yoga flow, notice if the mind has a lot to say. It might say things like, I can't do this, I'm bored, or What am I going to eat for lunch? If it does, that's fine. Your job is to simply become aware of it. Yoga is the union of breath, body, and spirit. The more we bring awareness to all three, the more we lessen the grip of the ego.

This next yoga sequence adds on nicely to the sun salutations on page 67. I encourage you to focus on your breath as you move through this flow. Notice if the ego pops in during the practice. When it does, come back to the breath and keep going. Keep recommitting to the next inhale and come back to the present moment.

LUNGE FLOW

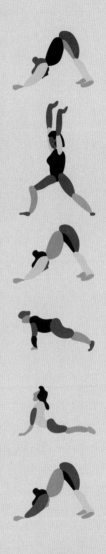

1. Begin in downward dog.

2. Step your right foot forward to a lunge.

3. Bring your arms over your head as you breathe in. Stay here for three breaths. Notice the reactions in the mind.

4. Step back into downward dog.

5. Come forward into high plank.

6. Lower to the floor, lowering your knees if you need to.

7. Come up into cobra pose.

8. Exhale and move back into downward dog.

9. Repeat the sequence, this time stepping your left foot forward.

(Repeat, stepping opposite foot forward)

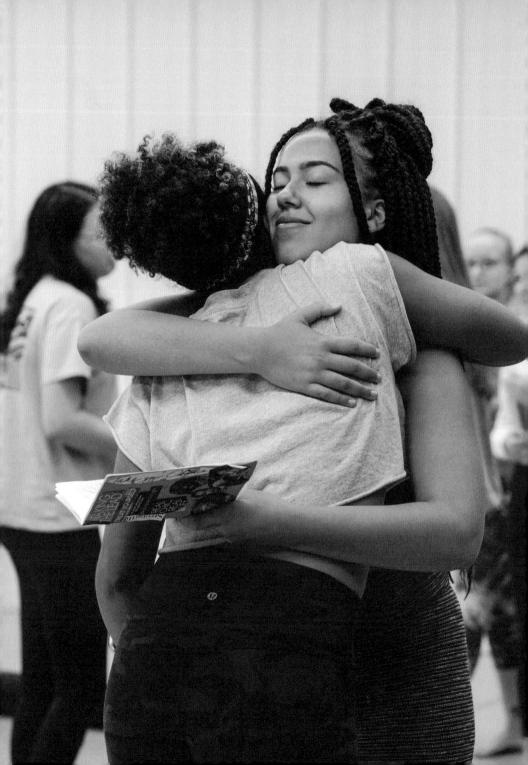

YOUR MIND IS LIKE A GARDEN

Like a garden, our minds are something we need to constantly tend to; otherwise, they can overgrow with egocentric thoughts. You have to keep watering your mind with powerful thoughts and weeding it of disempowering ones. This is to support your mental health. It's normal to have bad days and to go through hard times, but practices like meditation, breathing exercises, and yoga asana can help you to move through some of the heaviness that tougher moments bring.

The world is challenging enough—we do not need our mental state to also be a war zone. Thinking is inevitable and an inescapable truth of our existence, so learning how to moderate our minds is the key. This won't happen in an instant—that's why I've offered various practices like yoga, meditation, and journaling—but over time you will get better at creating a new reality for yourself.

143

JOURNAL

One of my favorite practices for getting out of any negative thought spirals is writing them down and flipping them. On a sheet of paper, draw two columns. In one, write down all the ugly, dark, negative, self-deprecating thoughts that are present in your brain, using "I am" statements. Don't be afraid to let it rip. Get all the awful things up there onto your paper. Then, in the second column, write down the exact opposite of each negative statement.

For example:

I am stupid. ➤ *I am wise and deeply intuitive.*
No one likes me. ➤ *I attract the right friends for me.*
I am a failure. ➤ *I am learning the right lessons
  to help me succeed.*
I hate my body. ➤ *I am learning to love myself as I am.*

This exercise allows us to address the thoughts, get them out, and change them into something we can actually work with. But something to keep in mind: It's important to choose a reframing statement that feels good to you and that feels doable. Create something that feels inspiring and real that will give you freedom from the negativity.

I do this exercise often when I am feeling stuck in my own self-sabotaging cycle. I use the new mantras I've created by repeating them to myself throughout the day, writing them in my journal each day, or posting them on my bathroom mirror.

YOUR TURN.

*We can
change our
minds.
We do have
the power
to shift.
It is safe to
feel good.
It is our
birthright
to feel.*

the power
of your heart

"My sensitivity is
a superpower.
I am not afraid of
my emotions."

—Abigail, 19,
VANCOUVER,
BRITISH COLUMBIA

04

LOLA

It is midweek at the Girlvana Spring Break retreat, and we gather in the yoga space in our usual circle. I lead a meditation to ground everyone in their bodies and to center us all in our hearts. The energy is serene, and there is trust in the room. Once we are all breathing in unison, I instruct everyone to reach out and find the hands beside them. As we inhale, we breathe into our hearts, and as we exhale, we squeeze each other's hands a little tighter. We are creating connection and a brave space for us all to exist in. "Bring all of you here," I say to everyone. "Here, you don't have to hide yourself. All parts of you are welcome." After five minutes of creating this safe space together, we open our eyes and look at each other. We take a moment with each person in the room to really see them and acknowledge them. It is a silent *I got you*, in the form of meeting eyes. I call this a "spiritual cheers"—like clinking your glasses together in celebration but using meaningful eye contact instead.

I give everyone a piece of paper and instruct them to write down their answers to the statement *If you really knew me, you would know that* . . . They don't need to write their names down; this will be anonymous. We crumple up all the pieces of paper and put them in the center of the circle. Then we each take one of the balls of paper. We close our eyes and take one collective, deep breath. Then we begin.

One by one each girl reads out the words of another girl. After each person shares, we pause and take a deep breath together before continuing. We don't know whose paper is whose, and it doesn't matter. What is important is that we give space for everyone's words to be listened to with love.

If you really knew me, you would know that . . .

"I have to hold it together for my mom after the divorce. I have to parent her. There is no one to be strong for me."

Inhale. Exhale.

"I puke after every meal because I hate my body and I don't know how to stop."

Inhale. Exhale.

"I am terrified of hooking up with anyone because of being molested as a kid."

Inhale. Exhale.

"I am gay and I am terrified to tell my parents."

Inhale. Exhale.

"I tried to kill myself last year and ended up in the hospital."

Inhale. Exhale.

"I had an abortion and I feel ashamed about it."

Inhale. Exhale.

"I don't think I have ever liked myself a day in my life."

Inhale. Exhale.

"I cut myself so I can punish myself for being stupid."

Inhale. Exhale.

"I was raped at a party and I'm afraid no one will ever love me."

Inhale. Exhale.

This circle is immensely raw. We've all spoken. There are lots of tears. Holding hands once again, we close our eyes and we breathe deeply. We transmute the suffering into love. We breathe in each other's stories and, as we breathe out, we free each other.

Most of us have never been in a more truthful space, a space where we can share our deepest secrets without having anyone turn their backs or judge us. In this space, we are held in our own truth and we are loved and accepted for who we are. In this space, we work together to witness our pain and suffering and free each other, simply by listening. It is the most sacred place I have ever known.

After the exercise, we break for free time and everyone runs to put their swimsuits on. We head to the ocean to jump in the cold water. There is a liberated excitement as we make our way down to the shore, wrapped in blankets and with arms wrapped around each other. We approach the water's edge with our air-dried tears. As everyone mentally prepares themselves to jump into the water on this chilly March day, Lola hangs behind.

Lola is fourteen, and she is still crying from the exercise. She is astonished at what everyone shared in that circle. Wrapped in a wool blanket, she looks at me, her teeth chattering. She looks awestruck and wild in her eyes. She tells me that she had no idea anyone other than her had felt those things, or had those things happen to them, at least no one she knows. She tells me through her hiccups and tears that, for the first time in her life, she feels free. She tells me which story was hers from the circle, and that she can't believe that people will still love her even though she tried to take her own life. She tells me she wants to live. And, for the first time in a long time, she is ready to live. She tells me about the weight that has been lifted from her heart. I give Lola a big hug, and anyone who has not already jumped into the water screaming like a charging warrior comes in for a group hug. "We love you, Lola!" we all sing. Then we rip off our blankets and join the rest of the group in the freezing cold ocean.

My goal with this exercise is to meet the source of our shame and hurt and speak it out loud, giving it permission to be released. The exercise proves that we are not alone, and once we all know each other in this personal way, we can love each other even more deeply. Our vulnerability allows us to pluck the pain from the body. It connects and relates us to others. It helps us find deep compassion for the people around us and, I believe, heals us as a collective.

THE HEART

This chapter is all about our hearts. Our hearts are a door-way to understanding our emotions. In the next few pages, I want to explore how, if we take the time to feel them fully, our emotions can empower us—and how they can hurt us if we choose to ignore them.

I think of human emotions as being like the weather. Sometimes we feel a thick fog or a light drizzle of rain, and other times we feel a complete thunderstorm, with lightning and a heavy downpour, within us. Many girls are taught that they have to act like sunshine all the time. A light drizzle every now and again is okay, but nothing too noisy. Most of us have internalized this message so deeply that when our storms come, we don't know what to do with them. We feel either panic or avoidance, because it can be a scary thing to feel our emotions. Does anyone really teach us how to ride out these storms? If we are too emotional, people may label us "crazy" or "unstable." It feels easier to pack up those emotions and shove them back down.

But if we do that, where do our emotions go? When you're feeling sad, angry, scared, or hurt, what helps you feel better?

NUMB OR RUN

When we are feeling big emotions, sometimes, to cope, we find ways to avoid having to face them. For example, if someone breaks your heart, or tells you they don't want to be friends with you, chances are you won't want to sit with the rejection and pain. You'd probably rather feel anything else than the weight of those emotions. So what do you do? In my own lived experience and from years of hearing from teens, I've learned dealing with big emotions can often involve numbing or running.

Numbing could be anything from drinking alcohol or drug use to cutting, starving yourself, binge eating, hooking up, or getting obsessive about external validation through social media. You see, when the emotions get really big, like a tsunami coming towards you, the urge to run away from them is all-encompassing. Of course it is! Why would we want to stay and feel the power of whatever those feelings are?

When we run, we keep ourselves hyper-distracted by something else as a way to be too busy to feel. This could look like obsessing over your schoolwork or job, or focusing a lot on your weight or exercise routine. At first, it can feel like you're winning the race against your emotions.

But regardless of how hard you try, your feelings will have a way of surfacing. Ignored feelings can end up being misdirected into anger towards someone else. Liza Palmer, author of *Conversations with the Fat Girl*, has said, "Angry is just sad's bodyguard."

Anger can often be a mask for what is really going on. Do you ever feel agitated, irritable, or like you have a short fuse, especially with the people you love? It could be that there is some unmet sadness in your heart that needs tending to. Instead of the obsessive behaviors of trying to distract or numb yourself, there is another solution. I will warn you that it is not always pretty, or perfect or easy. In fact, it is mostly messy and scary—but it works.

FEEL TO HEAL

Running or numbing our emotions can be exhausting. It can feel incredibly heavy to drag these unfelt feelings around in our day-to-day life, and it takes a lot of energy to constantly be dodging our innermost feelings.

In his book *The Untethered Soul*, Michael A. Singer writes about a thorn in your forearm that directly touches a nerve. Every time the thorn gets touched, it's very painful. So painful, in fact, that all of your choices are now shaped by the goal of keeping the thorn untouched. You can't sleep well, you avoid people getting close to you, you do everything to avoid the pain. Eventually, you end up building protective devices to shelter this thorn so no one and nothing will touch it. The obvious answer, of course, would be to pull the thorn out and let your arm bleed and heal so you can get back to your life, but if we look deeper into this metaphor, we can see why that may be hard.

We often choose to protect the "thorn" because we don't want to go through the pain of pulling it out. However, eventually, the protection we must create to keep the thorn safe and untouched begins to impact every other part of our lives—our activities, our relationships, and our experiences. Our energy becomes misplaced in trying to protect the thorn (our emotions) instead of just pulling it out and bleeding (feeling) so that we can heal.

PERMISSION TO FEEL

This concept of feeling our feelings can be foreign to a lot of us. We haven't necessarily been trained to feel or taught how to sort and make sense of our emotions. Society tends to encourage us to paint over our emotions. *Just smile! Chin up!* The repercussions of trying to remain positive all the time can make us feel as though we really must be broken.

But how do we actually address what is upsetting us? The first step is to give yourself permission to feel your feelings.

Remember in chapter two, when I told you the story of my break-in? That is this concept at play: making a safe space for yourself to get quiet and listen to what is going on inside your heart. Can you name the feeling? Where does it live? What is it saying?

HOW TO FEEL

This is a practice that can be done anytime to connect to your feelings. It is a series of queries that can help you identify the heaviness, loneliness, or confusion you may be feeling. When we can identify the feeling, we are better able to tend to it and release it. The more time we spend doing this, the easier it becomes to be with our emotions.

1. Find a safe and quiet place to be. Try your bedroom, or a place in nature.

2. Give yourself permission to feel by repeating to yourself, *It is safe for me to feel.*

3. Deepen your breath and notice if there is any resistance in your body. Are there any areas that feel tight in your chest or belly?

4. Ask your body to reveal to you any thorns that might need attention.

5. Feel the emotions that arise by breathing deeper. Imagine breathing into the emotion, meeting the feeling with your breath.

6. Can you name the emotion?

7. If the emotion could speak, what would it say?

8. Where does this emotion live inside of your body?

9. Stay with the feeling as long as the emotion needs you, and continue to breathe.

10. Thank the emotion for revealing itself to you.

IT'S OKAY TO CRY

Raise your hand if someone has ever said to you, "Stop crying;" "Please don't cry;" or "Are you crying *again?*" These comments are part of a narrative that I, like so many people, have heard my whole life. I have one rule when I lead yoga retreats and it is to *never apologize for crying.* When we apologize for crying, we are implying that we are ashamed of our own emotions and that our tears are unacceptable, especially in public spaces ... and especially around men. Well, we have been apologizing for our emotions our whole lives, and it is time to stop.

VULNERABILITY IS OUR SUPERPOWER

I see vulnerability as bravery. It takes a lot of courage to express how we are feeling, but it can also be really freeing. Think of Lola's realization after the "If you really knew me" activity. We aren't meant to keep all of these emotions trapped inside our bodies. So it's crucial for us to find brave spaces to share what is in our hearts.

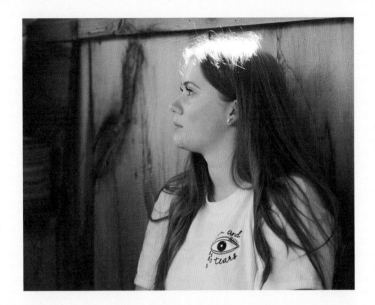

Emotions
are energy
in motion.

159

I also see vulnerability as a way to connect. When all the girls share together at Girlvana it allows them to see that they are not alone. Sharing something tough can be a gateway for someone else's own healing or acceptance.

THE MOVEMENT OF EMOTIONS

It can feel like the sweetest release to cry, and that's because crying actually does relieve stress. Cortisol, the stress hormone, is released from your body through the act of crying. Have you ever cried for a while and then slept like a baby?

Well, it turns out that the release of cortisol through our tears makes us feel calmer. It seems silly to say sorry for relieving our stress, doesn't it?

Emotions are simply energy in motion. So when we stuff down our emotions because we don't want to feel them, they will eventually gain momentum and blow up, arriving as an angry outburst, a breakdown, or a panic attack.

This is why I really started to fall in love with yoga. The physical movement and breath of yoga gave me a way to unearth and move some of my stuffed-down feelings. Yoga gave me tools to not be so scared of what I was experiencing. I could move my body and breathe deeply, and I would always feel so much lighter. When we address our darkness, we move through it. When I teach, I often say, "Come as you are." You don't need to be perfect or happy or calm. In fact, come with your heavy feelings, your sorrow, your grief. Emotions need space to be felt and released. I see exhaled breaths and tears and deep stretches as a powerful way to move our emotions. And our yoga mats never judge. I've always found that the breath and postures always end up being the perfect medicine.

IT'S OKAY TO BE ANGRY

In addition to not having spaces to cry and to express sadness, girls often don't get permission to be angry either. The expectation that we always be happy can prevent us from feeling our true feelings. Growing up, I felt like boys had more space than I did to express anger with their bodies and voices, through sport and roughhousing. I see a lot of my teens come to Girlvana with trapped anger or rage. What are we supposed to do with all of the unrealistic expectations put upon us?

When we start to get in touch with how we feel through yoga and meditation, we are often surprised to see that there is some rage there—that we are mad about all the inequalities and injustices in this world. Some days we *can't* just slap on a smile. Some days we *can't* stomach living up to the ridiculous notions of society, peers, and parents. Sometimes we *can't* just journal and breathe deeply. Sometimes we need to scream! And guess what? That is perfectly okay.

If you have come to a Girlvana retreat before, you might be familiar with two of our favorite exercises: screaming and punching the ocean, and scream-singing an emotional song during yoga. The reason I invite these types of practices into the retreat is so that we all have a safe way to let our anger go. Have you ever let out a scream with no one around? Have you ever belted a song at the top of your lungs with a bunch of other people willing to do the same? Have you ever used your voice like that? It can be therapeutic. Screaming can cleanse the heart. It can dispel heaviness. It can teach you how to use your voice with confidence.

So find something that helps you free the anger, whether it's dancing hard to a song you love, boxing, punching a pillow, or going for a run.

The only
way out
is through.

FISTS OF ANGER

Another really cool way to feel and dispel anger in a safe and useful way is through a breath exercise called "fists of anger." This exercise comes from the Kundalini yoga tradition and was taught to me by a teacher called Guru Jagat. It's an exercise I use with teens all the time. It's especially helpful when you can't necessarily find the words to express yourself.

1. Sit cross-legged, with a tall spine.

2. Tuck your thumbs in and make fists
   with your hands.

3. Bend at the elbows , keeping your
   forearms parallel to the floor, and
   begin to move your arms forward and
   back over your head, at a quick pace.
   The arms remain bent as you alternate
   them forward (in front of your body)
   and back (above your head and behind
   your body).

4. As you switch your arms, breathe
   through your mouth in short exhales
   (see breath of fire, page 134).

5. Really let yourself go here. Breathe
   with intention and let your arms fly.

6. If any emotions bubble up, let
   them come.

7. Try this for two minutes at first,
   and work your way up to five.

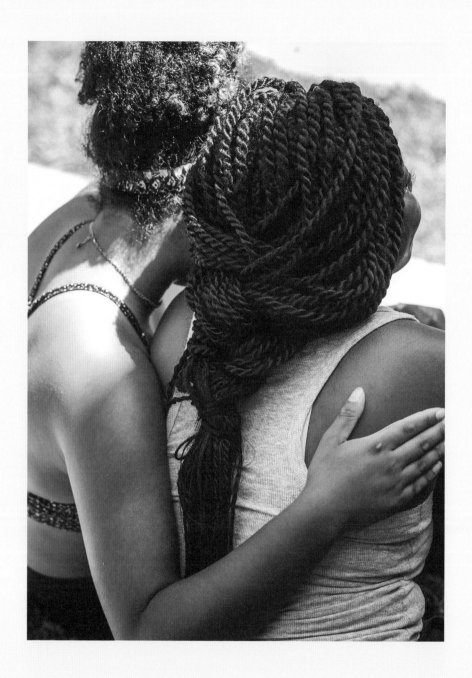

WHAT IS LOVE?

Girls are often conditioned to believe that love is something we have to earn. We are told we have to be good little girls in order for someone to love us. Look at Disney movies and fairy tales: it's always the prince that sweeps the girl off her feet and saves her—so long as she is beautiful and plays by the rules.

When I was younger, love felt like something you had to wait around for. If you just put all your effort into looking and acting a certain way and being a "cool girl," then someone might come along and choose you. But what if love doesn't come around? Does that mean you're not worthy of it? I was seeing this in myself as well as in my friends: our very sense of self-worth was teetering on whether or not someone liked us back. Why were we waiting around for someone else to determine our value? Why was our worthiness wrapped up in how someone else saw us? I had no idea that it was up to me to determine myself worthy.

165

DISCOVERING SELF-LOVE

Often when we think of love, we think of romantic or familial love. Rarely do we think of loving ourselves. No one told me that love wasn't about someone else choosing me—it was about choosing myself. *That* is my definition of self-love. When you choose yourself, you always have you to come home to. And when you focus on the love you have for yourself, you don't have to go out in the world, searching for someone to love you—that person will show up. Your worthiness is your decision to make.

You will experience first loves and first heartbreaks. There will be moments that will make you question your worth or people who will try to tell you who you are. In these times, stay strong and remember the value you bring to the world. Stand firmly in your "I am" statement (page 50) and know who you are. Dating or being in a relationship is not worth changing, hiding, or shrinking yourself for. Always choose yourself, and always remember your worth. Do not let anyone define it for you, or take it from you.

The same can be said about friendships. If you feel like you have to shrink yourself to fit into your friendships, these people are not your friends. Pretending to be someone you are not is a dangerous thing. It diminishes your spirit, and it strips you from your intuition and your heart.

Navigating relationships with romantic partners, friends, and even family can be tricky as a young adult, but the cool thing is that when we choose ourselves, we attract others who honor and uplift us. When we show up as who we truly are, other people who are doing the same will come into our lives (and faking who we are will bring us fake friends). The people around us are reflections of who we are. When we have generous, loving friends, chances are we exude those same qualities! If we have toxic, harsh, and gossipy friends, it can show us the places within ourselves that we need to heal. By choosing to work on ourselves instead of trying to fix others, we redirect our love inward and attract that same kind of love outwardly.

CHOOSING YOURSELF FIRST

It can be a scary thing to choose yourself, especially when people around you don't get it. Chances are, you not choosing yourself has been working for other people in your life. When you give others your sole attention, it feels good for them. When you don't love yourself, they are getting something from you. So when you recognize this and make the switch to valuing yourself instead of getting your self worth from others, it may piss people off. It will shift the dynamic of your relationships—and you may even see that some relationships no longer fit you. I hear this all the time from the teens I work with—that they no longer fit into the puzzle of their friend group or partnership.

When you begin the journey of loving yourself, it starts to become evident that there could be people in your life who are toxic. Whether they make you feel unsafe, unheard, or undervalued, you may find that you need to create space away from them in order to support your overall well-being and health. This is completely normal as you grow up and into yourself.

I know it's scary, especially in high school, but it is okay to outgrow friendships and relationships. When we have history with people, it can be really hard to say goodbye. Below is a template I have created and shared over the years for anyone who is looking to get out of a friendship. I created this template to help you move forward, if or when you need it. Whether you say or send this, it can be a really good way to get clear on how you feel.

HOW TO BREAK UP WITH A FRIEND

Dear _____,

I am currently working on supporting myself physically, mentally, and emotionally. In order to do that, I need to take some time and space away from our friendship. In the past I haven't always felt (*fill in the blank:* supported, cared for, understood, seen for who I truly am). Please respect my need for space as I choose myself, my health, and my worth. I truly wish you the best.

Sincerely,

_____

DON'T LET ANYONE STEAL YOUR ENERGY

Being able to voice when something is not serving you and take action is an essential part of self-love. When we are able to recognize who in our life is supporting us and who is not, we become freer. Toxic people can steal our precious energy, and you are too valuable and too special to have someone in your life who makes you feel otherwise. If you don't feel supported, seen, and loved by your friends, then it is time to let them go. The third yama, asteya, relates to this. Asteya asks us to look at who and what is stealing our time. Do you have anyone in your life right now who you feel takes up too much space in your schedule or even in your head? Does that person steal your energy, your truth, or your ability to feel good about yourself?

CHOSEN FAMILY

Relationships can get even trickier when it comes to family, especially when we are young and have to live in a dynamic that we don't always have control over. Perhaps your family, or legal guardians, don't fully understand you or make you feel seen or heard. Perhaps they have hurt or abused you, or failed to show up in a way that supports who you are and the choices that you make. In our quest to know ourselves and define who we are, it is often our families that are the most triggering.

If this is something you experience, I would encourage you to seek out a chosen family, a network of people who love you for you, and who make you feel safe and seen, especially if you're not getting that at home. Chosen family has helped me and so many of the teens I know get through incredibly hard times. We need people, even if it is one person, who care to witness us as we move through life.

There have been many times when I have used some form of the friendship breakup template with my family to create boundaries when I needed to protect my emotions.

Fill your
own cup
first.

As young women, we have been taught to be flimsy with our
boundaries, to be appeasable, easygoing, and open. But creating boundaries is actually an act of self-love. Do not shy
away from standing firm in and declaring what you need.
Keep people around who respect your boundaries, not
those who trample all over them. Your job is to take care
of yourself first. Fill your own cup first. People who respect
and honor your boundaries are worth keeping around.

EMPOWERMENT FOR ALL

170

My hope is that you are beginning to see that you deserve to
take care of you. That you are worthy of your own love. That
you have value beyond what others think about you. That
you can choose and define your worth. This is the beginning
of empowerment. When you feel powerful with love of the
self, then you can help others do the same. When we fill our
own cups with love they spill over and fill others'.

Our self-discovery journeys are very personal. They are
winding roads of light and dark that bring us back home
to our true selves. Once I began to recognize that I was a
powerful person and I didn't have to wait around for love,
I wanted to shout it from the rooftops! It is why I created
Girlvana—I wanted to share this information. I wanted others to fill their cups with self-love.

It's important to remember that none of the tools—
the breathing exercises, the yoga, the meditations—we are

learning will ever be powerful if we don't share them with others and use them to help elevate one another, especially other women. Real power is about helping others, and it is joyous and glorious. It is one of the most rewarding things we can do. It is something we must do.

We have to acknowledge that historically women have been pitted against each other, and I believe this is a way to keep us small and keep us busy. Consider the narratives we grew up with in movies, TV shows, and books. We rarely saw girls liking and supporting each other; stories were generally centered around girls competing for a job, a guy, or a friendship, or making a decision about who was the most beautiful or popular.

The more time we spend comparing ourselves to one another and putting down other females, the less likely we are to pay attention to what is going on with those who hold power. Adrienne Rich, an American poet, essayist, and feminist, wrote, "The connections between and among women are the most feared, the most problematic, and the most potentially transforming force on the planet." This is a very powerful statement and I believe it! There are so many injustices in this world, and things have to change. Our generation's revolution can come from us not trying to take each other out but rather upholding each other and moving each other forward. It is time for us to love ourselves boldly and connect, and encourage others to do the same. I am especially passionate about women lifting one another up as it pertains to privilege. It's not enough that we just

171

Creating boundaries is an act of self-love.

uphold those who speak, act, and look like us; we need to be listening to and loving *all* women, especially those who hold less privilege in the world.

WHAT IS PRIVILEGE?

Privilege is defined as a special right, advantage, or immunity granted or available only to a particular person or group.

White privilege is defined as the unearned, mostly unacknowledged social advantage white people have over other racial groups simply because they are white.

White supremacy, as defined by yoga teacher and social justice activist Michelle Cassandra Johnson, is an ideology and belief system that is based on a hierarchy of constructed racial categorizations in which white is at the top and Black is at the bottom. She goes on to say in her book, *Skill in Action*, that "white supremacy is a belief system that perpetuates the idea that white is superior."

White women need to listen to, support, and elevate Black people, Indigenous people, and other people of color (BIPOC) who have not had the same allowances they've had. This isn't to say that some white people haven't had hard lives, but we haven't had hard lives *because* we are white.

Our feminism must include all women, period. If feminism is not intersectional, it is just white supremacy. We must unearth our unconscious biases and see that all women deserve a seat at the table. Sometimes for white women that might mean stepping back and putting someone else

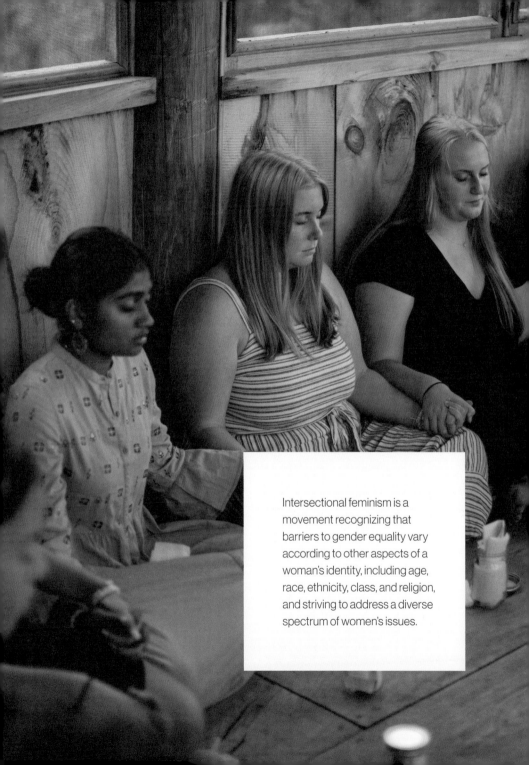

Intersectional feminism is a movement recognizing that barriers to gender equality vary according to other aspects of a woman's identity, including age, race, ethnicity, class, and religion, and striving to address a diverse spectrum of women's issues.

forward. This is another way in which the yama asteya functions. It asks us to look at where we might be unaware of our own privilege and how we could be stealing acknowledgment or opportunities from BIPOC.

Our singular goal is not to just "win" at this thing called life—because we all know no one gets out alive—but for *all* of us to make it to the finish line. In order to do that we must see that not everyone shares the same starting line—in fact, some are not even on the field. People who hold a lot of privilege often are blind to the fact that so many others do not have access to health care, a proper education, or job security due to discrimination based on race, gender, or sexual identity. People with privilege, particularly white privilege, think they are constantly hitting home runs, but they were starting on third base.

HOW TO USE OUR PRIVILEGE

In order to use our privilege for good, we must understand our social location. *Social location* refers to the advantages we have been given due to our race, gender, social class, body ability, sexual orientation, religious beliefs, and where we live in the world. To be clear, the world is set up to support white, able-bodied, straight, cisgender people. Do you fall into one of these categories? Can you take the unearned advantages that come with your position and amplify those who do not have the same allowances and safety in this world? For a white person, this could look like sharing the work of young Black activists on the frontlines of the Black Lives Matter movement. If you are straight, could you educate yourself on the LGBTQ+ community and see if you can donate time, money, or resources? If you are cisgender, can you learn about the struggles of trans people to help to ensure that they are represented and protected in your schools?

Privilege is, in a lot of ways, just unearned access to power and resources. If we have this access just because of who we are and where we come from, it's important that we consider what we can do to help others who do not have it.

Here are some other ways to use your privilege:

175

+ If you get a ride to an activity each week from a family member, could you offer a ride to someone who can't make it there on time because they don't have the same transportation options as you?

+ If you have access to an abundance of fresh and healthy food at home, perhaps you could bring it to school and share with others who do not?

+ Do you have a platform, like as school president or captain of a team? Could you make sure that your teams and clubs are including Black people and other people of color? If you don't have this platform, can you speak up and ask that activities, teams, and clubs be more inclusive?

- Do you have extra clothing that you don't wear that someone else could use? Can you donate it or share it with teammates, neighbors, or classmates?

- Can you talk to your parents about how they can use their privilege in their life and at their jobs?

- Can you lobby to get gender-neutral bathrooms in your school?

Take a few minutes to think about the privileges you have that you did not necessarily earn. How could you give to, support, or amplify those who may not have the same advantages? I implore you to keep waking up to what you have and truly seeing what others do not. Taking a look at what has been freely given to us and using it not just to benefit ourselves but to uplift others is what is going to change our world. My friend and fellow yoga teacher Dr. Chelsea Jackson Roberts says, "We cannot compartmentalize our liberation." To me this means that yoga is meant to free us—our minds, our hearts, our bodies—but it does not stop with just us. We must work to liberate us all.

The aim of Girlvana is to teach you how to love and liberate yourself so you can go out and truly love and liberate the world.

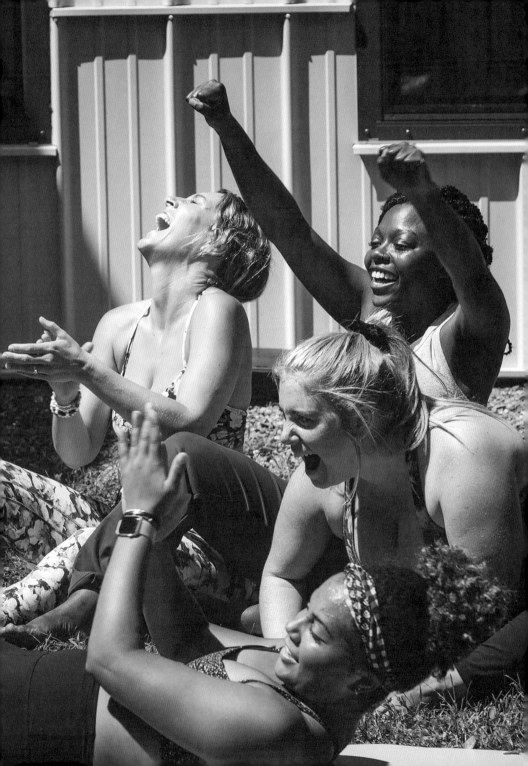

SELF-LOVE MEDITATION

This simple meditation is designed for you to be there for yourself and be the generator of your own love when you need it the most. The more we practice cultivating love for ourselves and showing up for ourselves, the more we can help empower those around us.

Remember that you are whole—you do not need to be fixed.

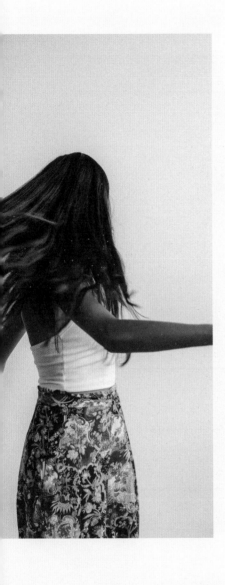

1. Lie down on your back.

2. Take the soles of your feet together and let your knees fall out to the sides.

3. Place one hand on your belly and the other on your heart and close your eyes.

4. Begin to inhale into your hands, feeling your belly and chest expand.

5. Exhale, relaxing deeper into the floor.

6. As you continue inhaling and exhaling, let the sensation of love fill your entire body. Imagine the feeling of love spreading through your head, heart, and belly.

7. Imagine breathing love in and breathing love out.

8. Remember that filling ourselves up with love will help us love others.

9. Keep breathing love in and out for up to five minutes.

179

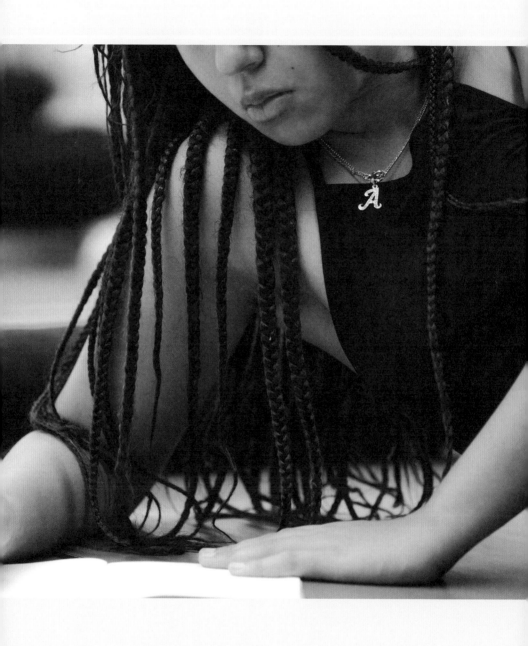

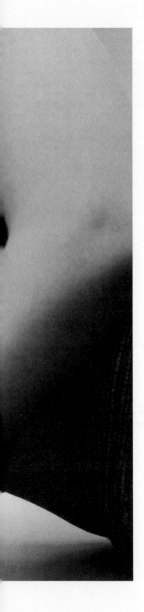

THE PRACTICE OF FEELING
YOUR FEELINGS FLOW

The sequence on the next page is all
about feeling our strength as we meet
our challenges. In it is a new pose called
warrior. Warrior poses are tough, and
they're supposed to be! In this pose,
we are meant to stay with the intensity.
Remember that yoga is a practice, and
when we can practice working through
a challenging moment in a pose, it can
help us do the same thing in life.

This sequence can be tacked onto the
previous chapters' or be done on its own.

181

Self-love takes time and practice. Be gentle with yourself if you forget or get lost; this love is always here, waiting for you to return. You can always come back home.

182

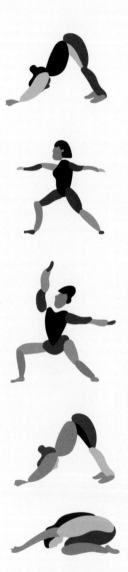

(Repeat, stepping opposite foot forward)

A PRACTICE IN STRENGTH

1. Come to downward dog.

2. Step your right foot forward and align your right knee over your ankle. Spin the back foot flat.

3. Reach your arms into a T shape. This pose is called warrior II.

4. As you hold the pose, keep the bend in your right knee. You will feel a burn, and instead of ignoring it or wishing it would go away, be with it.

5. Reverse your warrior pose by taking your left hand to your left leg and reaching your right arm to the sky. This should feel like a side bend in your spine. Hold for a breath or two.

6. Windmill your hands back to the floor and step back to downward dog.

7. Repeat steps 1 to 6, this time stepping forward with your left foot.

8. End in child's pose.

183

Sometimes we all need to be reminded that our worth is not wrapped up in someone else's opinion or tied to society's expectations. If you are feeling drained by the need to have someone love you or validate your existence, this flow will be really helpful to you.

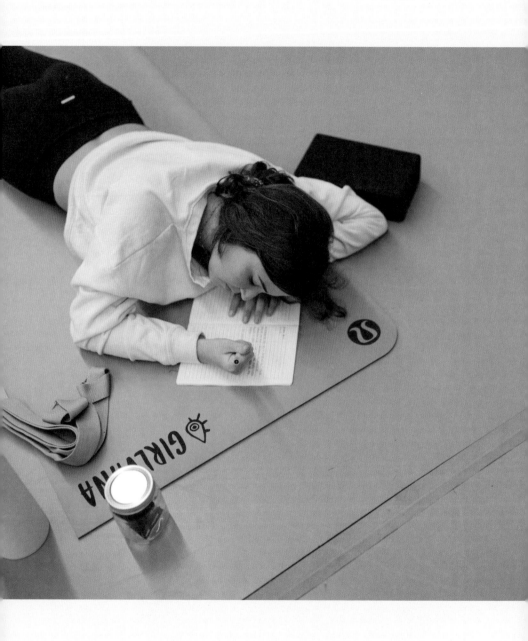

JOURNAL

Years ago, my friend Jian Pablico introduced me to this statement: *If you really knew me, you would know that . . .* The idea is to truthfully answer something about yourself that is hidden inside, perhaps something that feels secretive or shameful. It is a way to speak your truth out loud and be met with love and compassion. If we peeked behind the curtain of your life, or truly saw beyond the mask, what would we discover about you?

This concept, of sharing a secret inside of us, began to take shape in a big way at my retreats. I loved that it sparked a deep dive into real talk faster than any question I had ever asked a group.

When we share what is really going on inside of us, the festering, secret pockets of shame that we carry are revealed, and we can move forward. I encourage you to do some journaling around this question on your own.

If you really knew me, you would know that . . .

YOUR TURN.

the power of
your soul

"Girlvana was the catalyst that started my journey into self love. It taught me that the woman I am is more than enough, and that no matter where I was in life, that's exactly where I was supposed to be."

—Avery, 16,
MADISON, WISCONSIN

05

TEDDY

Teddy is fifteen, and she tells me that every time she is with him something doesn't feel right. She can't explain it; it just feels off. We're sitting on the floor in the yoga studio after a Girlvana class. Her arms clutch her shins and tears sit heavy in her eyes, seconds from dropping. Teddy knows she should leave her boyfriend, but he keeps convincing her to stay. She tells me that he's often verbally abusive, that he makes her do sexual things she isn't ready to do, and that she doesn't like who she is becoming. She thought that he loved her, but she's starting to feel like this isn't love. Isn't love supposed to feel good? Isn't love supposed to make you feel like the best version of yourself? She asks me these questions earnestly. She can't make sense of it. He's popular and well liked; her friends think he's cool, and her parents seem to think he's a nice guy. She tells me he

Intuition is
the soul's way
of speaking.

always apologizes when he says something mean or pushes things too far. He always has a way of making it better, telling her that things will be different going forward. In her mind Teddy believes him, but today in yoga, something new began coming to the surface.

I ask her how she truly feels when she is with him, and she tells me she feels small, unlovable, ugly, and dumb. I ask her what it physically feels like in her body when he says mean things to her or forces her to go further than what she feels ready for. She explains the clenching in her stomach and the tightness in her throat. "It feels like the opposite of yoga," Teddy says.

"What would you like to feel in a relationship?" I ask her. "How would you like it to feel in your body?"

She says it feels like deep breaths. She feels spacious, and there is an ease. "When I really listened to my heart in the yoga practice today," she begins, "I heard it—or maybe it was my whole body—say, *Break up with him*." But now she's having a hard time deciphering the right answer.

I tell Teddy that what she is feeling is her intuition. We can often think ourselves into or out of any situation, but if we really want the truth, we must *feel*.

Teddy nods. "I've been feeling this way for a while," she admits.

"When was the first time you felt this way?" I ask.

"On our first date," she says. It was like there was always something not quite right, but she pushed those feelings away, convincing herself that it was cool to have a popular boyfriend and that it was her fault for not wanting to go further.

We keep talking, and suddenly Teddy is sure: It is time to prioritize herself and to listen to this gut feeling. It is time to break up with him.

Your intuition is often a feeling rather than a thought.

THE POWER OF INTUITION

In this chapter we are going to explore the concept of intuition, or *inner knowing*, and how that is different than the ego. Our default setting is often to listen to the ego before checking in with our intuition. However, whether we know it or not, our body is always sending us signals, and when we are able to direct our energy inwards, we can start to pick up on those messages that are beyond thought. The fourth yama, brahmacharya, teaches us moderation and to let go of external desires and go inward. When we go inward, we can hear our own wisdom.

Have you ever experienced a deep sense of knowing that something was either right or wrong, beyond any words or rationale? That's your intuition, appearing as a gut feeling. It's not of the mind, and it's not something that is born from thought.

When we make decisions purely from the mind, we consider a lot of external factors and expectations, which can be very exhausting and confusing. This can make us even more uncertain, because the mind has a way of holding up

193

Brahmacharya is the fourth yama, and it is defined as the highest and best use of our vital energy. It teaches us to not only look at where we are directing our energy, but also ask why (see page 35).

*Your intuition
is the ability
to understand
something
immediately,
without the need
for conscious
reasoning. Most of
us are not taught
to honor our
intuition—instead,
we're told to value
logic over feeling.
Then, when we
experience the
sensations of our
intuition, we
immediately go
to our thoughts to
try to justify our
response and talk
ourselves out of
the feeling.*

arguments for each side. But we've also learned that our thinking minds are not always telling us the truth. Yoga teaches that the intuition is an inner knowing; it is something that is alive within our bodies. The intuition doesn't consider thought; it simply has an immediate response to what it is witnessing.

You've probably felt your intuition before, but did you actually listen to it? When you don't check in with what it is that you want instead of just trying to please others, making even trivial decisions is challenging. Yoga can teach us how to tune in to our bodies and listen to the internal signals of what is actually going on within us. One of the most important things we can learn about our intuition is what our *yes* and *no* feel like inside us.

There have been so many times in my life where I have said yes when I meant no. This could be anything from deciding what to eat for dinner to a sexual advance. I've often heard from girls and women (and I've felt this myself) that our opinions don't hold value in society, that we often feel expected to comply. However, when we do that, we eventually lose our ability to advocate for ourselves. Learning how to use our intuition is not something we are taught in school. Neither is learning how to listen to those gut feelings and act upon them. We have to learn to listen on our own.

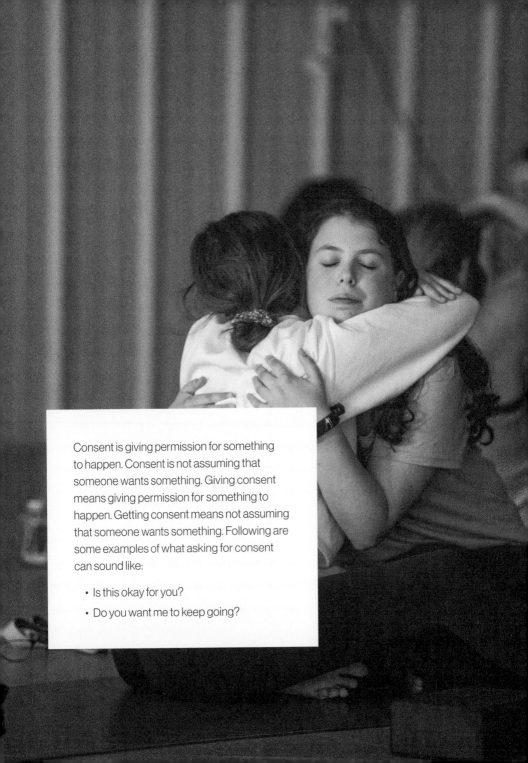

Consent is giving permission for something to happen. Consent is not assuming that someone wants something. Giving consent means giving permission for something to happen. Getting consent means not assuming that someone wants something. Following are some examples of what asking for consent can sound like:

- Is this okay for you?
- Do you want me to keep going?

CONSENT

Over time, as I used the self-awareness practices we've been discussing, I've learned what *yes* feels like in my body and what *no* feels like. For example, if I'm in a yoga posture and I feel like I'm pushing myself too far, I back off. Off the mat and in real life, I can feel my intuition in situations where I am overdoing it or pushing myself beyond what feels safe.

Knowing what *yes* and *no* feel like in your body is really important when it comes to consent in sex. Consent is sometimes viewed as a gray area, and we often carry a lot of shame and guilt around sexual interactions that we are uncomfortable with. I have heard from so many young women (and I've also experienced this!) who have woken up the morning after and asked themselves, *Did I actually want that to happen? Did I say yes?* Or they feel shame wondering why they didn't say no when it truly felt like a no in their bodies.

Obviously, the conversation about consent is not our sole responsibility; all genders have to be involved. We need to educate them. We all need to be in the practice of asking the question, "Is this okay with you?" And it's important to note that this is not a one-time question, but something to ask throughout any interaction with someone, especially if it is intimate. But we have to start by learning to ask ourselves, *Is this okay with me?* We need to be able to identify this within ourselves first so that we can better express ourselves and honor where we are at.

I understand that speaking your truth during a sexual interaction can be incredibly terrifying. I often hear from girls that they have sometimes let sexual interactions continue for fear of not being liked or for fear of making the other person feel bad. They prioritize others' comfort over their own.

You can start to identity your *yes* and your *no* by asking yourself these questions:

+ What does *yes* feel like in your body? What is the feeling, the sensation that you experience?

+ What happens when you feel *no*? Where do you sense the *no* in your body? How does it present in your body language, in the sound of your voice, in the way you sit, speak, or hold yourself?

When we can identify what our *yes* and *no* feel like, we can use that knowledge as our base for making decisions around food, friends, work, and ultimately all our life choices.

While we must stop saying yes when we mean no out of fear that we will disappoint others, we also must stop saying no to opportunities that actually feel like a yes to us. Sometimes self-doubt will kick in and say, *Who are you to do that?* or *Who do you think you are?* That voice will make us believe that we aren't talented, smart, or prepared enough for whatever is in front of us. It can also be terrifying to take the leap outside of our comfort zone because we're worried

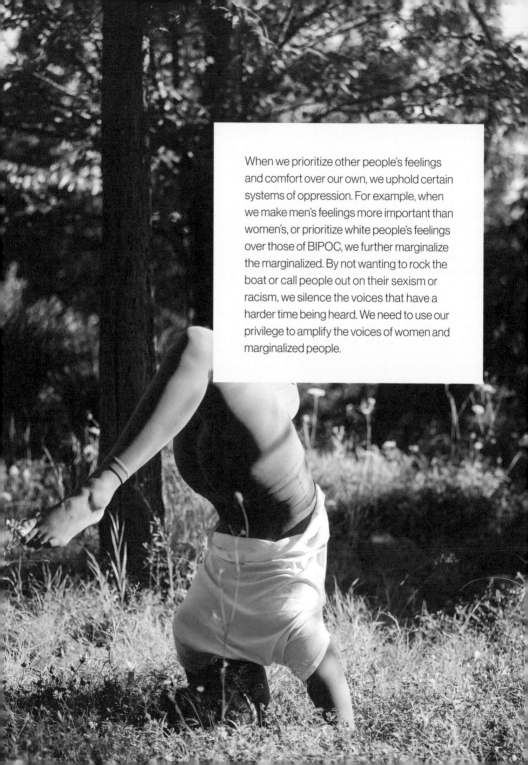

When we prioritize other people's feelings and comfort over our own, we uphold certain systems of oppression. For example, when we make men's feelings more important than women's, or prioritize white people's feelings over those of BIPOC, we further marginalize the marginalized. By not wanting to rock the boat or call people out on their sexism or racism, we silence the voices that have a harder time being heard. We need to use our privilege to amplify the voices of women and marginalized people.

about what others will say. In either of these instances, we need to be brave and say yes when it feels like a yes. We need to step more fully into this world!

Understanding what *yes* and *no* feel like in our bodies will ultimately guide us on our path, but remember that there is no such thing as the *right* path or the right way. Regardless of what we have been taught about success and the correct way to do things (eat, date, get a job, go to college), there is no right way—there is only *your* way. Your way will not look like anyone else's—not your parents', your teachers', or your friends'. It will be the one you carve out through your beliefs, gifts, and experiences.

We need you in this world. We need your unique gifts and talents. We need you to stop saying no when you mean yes.

199

SELF-CARE

Let's explore what it looks like to truly take care of ourselves. Self-care is crucial to our well-being; however, it's often touted as ways to feel good when you feel bad. Often it looks like things to buy and indulge in when you are feeling low. True self-care is the action of caring for ourselves each and every day. Of course it can be nice to use a bath bomb and a face mask, but a bath bomb and face mask are not necessary to take care of yourself—"things" are not what take care of you. The way you treat yourself, feed yourself, and rest yourself is what takes care of you.

*Ask yourself:
How am I?
How do I
feel? What
do I need to
support myself
right now?*

In the past I have looked to friends, family, and partners to take care of me. If I was upset, I would expect them to solve my problems for me. Over time I would start to feel let down when they didn't have the answers that I needed, or when they couldn't make me happy. I realize now that taking care of me, making me happy, wasn't their job.

It is your job to maintain your inner landscape. Yes, others can help and support and love you (community is very important), but at the end of the day it is how you treat yourself that matters most. From there, the friendships and relationships that arrive will be a direct reflection of how you feel about yourself. I encourage you to speak to and act towards yourself in a compassionate way as a form of self-care. I know that I can't charge my batteries or refuel my energy if I am still battling or shaming myself. Our energy is recharged from true care.

When we treat ourselves with care, we deepen the relationship we have with our capital-S Self. Everything comes back to this relationship, the one you have with yourself. Taking care of ourselves is not selfish, nor is it a luxury. It is a necessity—especially if we want to get out there and change the world. We need the energy to do so.

I also view self-care as a moment-to-moment inquiry to discover what you need. Create your own personal toolkit for self-care, so that when you are really struggling you can say, *Oh right! I can go for a walk, take five breaths, call a safe friend, drink a glass of water, play music, or take a nap.*

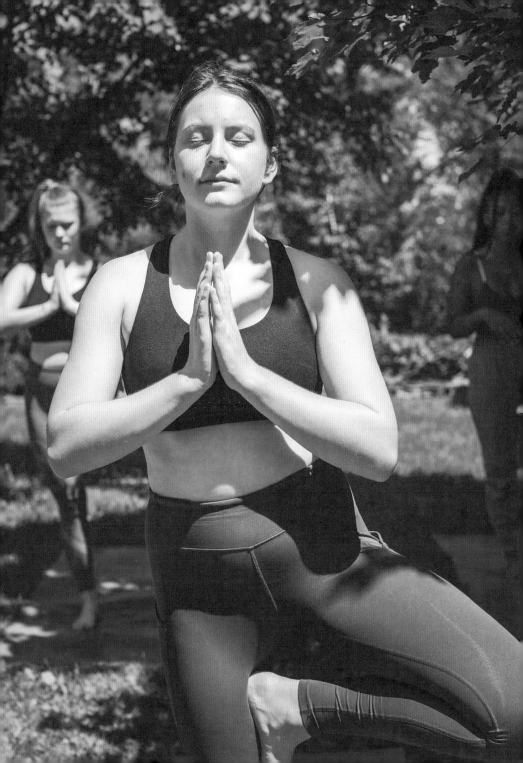

Remember that self-care doesn't have to cost anything. Choose things that are free and readily available for when you need them the most.

Here is a list of my favorite quick and free self-care tools—pulled together by some amazing teens I know—to shift you out of a funk.

SELF-CARE CHECKLIST

202

*Maintaining
your inner
landscape is
about directing
your precious
energy inward,
towards yourself,
instead of
towards external
distractions.*

- Water your plants
- Watch puppy videos on your phone
- Sit outside with your face to the sun
- Make a cup of tea
- Tell someone how you are feeling
- Light a candle and write in your journal
- Sing or yell in the car or shower
- Say no to plans and watch your favorite movie
- Wash your sheets and make your bed
- Go for a walk
- Draw
- Take a bath
- Make a vision board
- Listen to music
- Do a yoga flow
  (there are some good ones in this book!)
- Do a short meditation
  (this book has lots of those, too!)

I invite you to make your own list of things that you know will make you feel good and most like yourself when you're down. Whatever you end up doing, just make sure that you are doing it for yourself.

Practicing taking care of ourselves gets easier. Eventually, when we prioritize ourselves, it becomes more of a habit to check in and give ourselves what we need. Have the courage to walk towards what you need—and towards yourself.

The Girlvana movement is about taking care of yourself and then taking care of others. You are worth the time and effort it takes to slow down and regenerate yourself. We are not here to save the world, but we are here to change it. Your generation holds the future in its hands, and learning how to take care of yourself in order to change the world will be your superpower.

Make self-care your superpower.

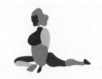

THE PRACTICE OF RELEASE

(Repeat, stepping opposite foot forward)

Our hips can be like emotional storage lockers. Unprocessed or suppressed feelings can get stuck in the body, and the hips tend to be the sticky spots for those things to hang out. This flow is designed to release stagnant energy in your hips. As you move through the postures, really focus on your breath and what it feels like to stay with any thoughts or sensations that are coming up for you.

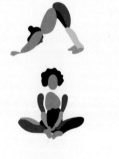

HIP-OPENING FLOW

1. From downward dog, place your right knee on the mat behind your right wrist and extend your left leg back behind you.

2. Place your forearms on the ground, stacking hands on top of each other, palms facedown.

3. Rest your head on your hands.

4. Take four to ten breaths here. You may feel a deep stretch in your hip. Make sure your knee isn't in pain.

5. Come back to downward dog.

6. Repeat steps 1 to 5, this time placing your left knee behind your left wrist.

7. Sit down on the mat and place the soles of your feet together. Let your knees fall open.

8. Draw your chin toward your chest and release your head. Don't worry if your head can't go that far.

9. Take four to ten breaths here.

10. Come to lie down on your back for savasana and relax for four to ten more breaths.

HONOR OR PUNISH

Self-care is not *what* you buy; it is *how* you listen. Listening to what we need and then providing it for ourselves is one of the most effective ways to practice self-care. If you are tired, take a nap. If you don't feel heard, write in your journal. Hungry? Eat. Overwhelmed? Breathe deeply.

When I am trying to determine what I need, I also like to ask myself, *Is this honoring or punishing?*

This is a powerful question to ask ourselves when we are making choices during the day about food, fitness, and even friends. For example, while eating well can honor our bodies, healthy food can also be used as a way to punish ourselves when we think we've been "bad." We may also use exercise in this way. It's important to be mindful of when something that should be incredibly honoring turns punishing instead.

Yes, it feels good to eat healthy food and move our bodies. I see these things contributing to overall well-being. But in the past, if the commitment to love myself wasn't there, I tended to use exercise and diet as weapons. Punishing myself for overeating meant doing a juice cleanse. Punishing myself for being lazy meant overdoing it at the gym.

When you come from a place of love for yourself, eating a delicious donut may actually be self-care for you versus eating a salad and hating yourself. Your body responds to intention. You cannot hate yourself into being healthy and well. The only way to be well is to do things out of love for yourself.

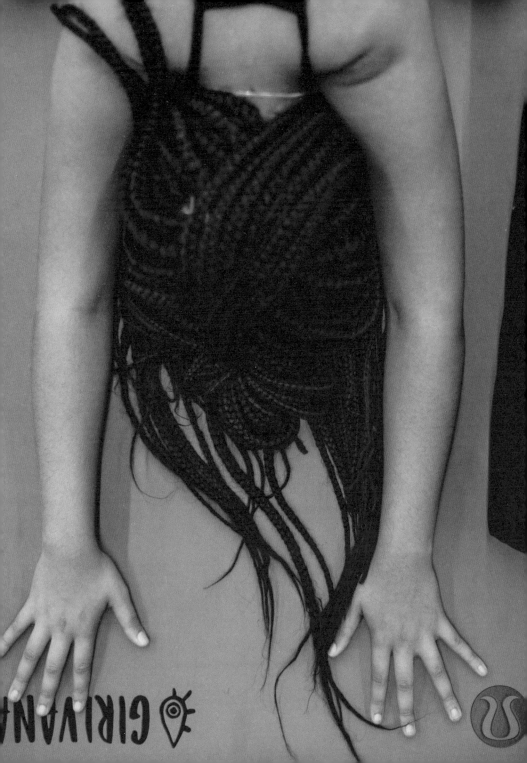

Make a list of your choices throughout the week and see what was honoring to your body and soul. Then, identify whether any of the decisions you made were based on a need to punish yourself.

HONOR	PUNISH
_____	_____
_____	_____
_____	_____
_____	_____
_____	_____
_____	_____
_____	_____
_____	_____
_____	_____

208

When I am supporting others, I ask them the same thing I ask myself: What do you need right now?

You may notice that some of your activities fall into both categories, and that's normal. Sometimes we use food to honor our bodies and other times we punish ourselves through bingeing, limiting, or purging. Sometimes we go to the gym to honor our bodies and feel our strength, while other times we use it to punish ourselves for eating too much over the weekend. You may also experience this with friends. Some friends will honor you, your choices, and who you are, while others may judge you or not get you. Being around them could feel punishing or harmful.

In asking yourself whether something is honoring or punishing, you will become aware of moments when you are being extra hard on yourself and don't need to be.

CONNECTING WITH THE MOON

The moon is associated with feminine energy. Just like us, it shines in its fullness but it also retreats and becomes new again. I look to the moon to remind myself of my power, my fullness, and my constant being and becoming. You may find that your emotions are heightened around the full moon. It could also be your bleeding time. (Some people find that their periods actually sync with the moon's cycles!)

One of my favorite self-care practices is setting and releasing intentions around the moon and its deeply powerful presence. I believe that as the moon becomes full, it offers deep brilliance to us. On the following pages are some of the rituals I like to perform around the moon's cycle.

The things that the wellness industry sells us don't actually take care of us unless our intentions behind using or consuming them are pure.

NEW MOON

The new moon represents a new phase. Think of it as an ushering in of new energy. This is a powerful time to set intentions and dream! This is a ritual that is meant to ground you and help you to get in touch with what you want. Make sure to have a journal or a notepad nearby.

I love to be in the bath and soak up all that I wish to create. I visualize it, speak it, and surrender into my dreams.

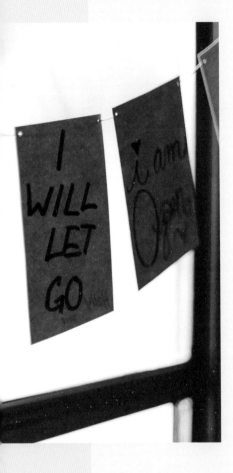

1. Find space to be alone, and take some time to get quiet. Meditation or a bit of movement will help you get yourself grounded.

2. Ask your heart what it truly desires right now. What are the dreams that are alive within you that you may not have the courage to speak about just yet?

3. Get clear on what these dreams are. How do they feel? What do they look like?

4. In your journal, write down one to five intentions for this fresh, new energy. Write your heart out.

5. Display your intentions where you can see them—your bedside, your bathroom mirror, your locker.

6. If you have access to a bathtub, make a bath! Fill it with salts, oils, flower petals, or crystals. Light candles and soak as you continue to dream up your manifestations. If you don't have a bathtub, a quick hot shower can also help soothe and relax you.

211

FULL MOON

The full moon has a different vibe from the new moon. This phase represents the end of a cycle, and it illuminates what needs to stay and what needs to go. This is a powerful time to take stock of where you are and to practice the art of letting go.

1. Light a candle or sit by a wood-burning fire or bon-fire. If you are using a candle, be sure to have a bowl of water close by. Always ask for permission before you do this.

2. Get quiet and thank the moon for her brilliance and power.

3. Write down what is no longer serving you: bad habits, negative thoughts, illness, toxic behaviors, relationship ties, ancestral pain, you name it. Where have you been hard on yourself? Where have you been beating yourself up? Punishing yourself?

4. Burn it! If you are using a candle, watch your paper burn and then drop it in the water. You can pour the water into the garden or simply toss it out.

5. Once your paper has burned, thank the moon again and sigh, taking deep releasing exhales.

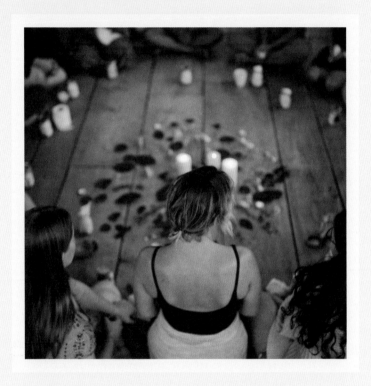

MEDITATION TO TAP INTO INTUITION

All of the teachings I'm sharing with you are meant to connect you more deeply with yourself and the world around you. Use this meditation when you are feeling confused about something or having a hard time making a decision—especially if you feel like you have too many opinions from others in your head. This meditation is designed to help you listen to your inner voice and trust your own truth. We will be using the concept of brahmacharya to direct our vital energy inwards and to release any sensory overload from others' opinions. Be sure to silence your phone and set up in a quiet area.

1. Get comfortable by sitting or lying down.

2. Close your eyes or soften your gaze.

3. Place your right hand on your belly and your left hand on your heart.

4. Breathe deeply into your belly and chest, feeling your hands rise and fall.

5. Ask yourself, *What am I feeling right now?* Continue to breathe deeply as your feelings come to the surface.

215

6. Now ask a question that you have been struggling with, something you do not necessarily have the answer to.

7. Take a pause, keep breathing, and let your intuition respond. You may notice that the mind wants to barge in and answer the question. Try to go deeper and see if you can *feel* the answer instead of thinking it.

8. Stay present and keep asking the question as much as you need to.

9. Let the answer rise up within you.

Your intuition will always be there to guide you. When you feel like you are taking the advice of too many people or that everyone has an opinion about what you should do, look within. Trust what you hear. Trust your intuition.

ALTERNATE NOSTRIL BREATHING

The Sanskrit name for alternate nostril breathing is *nadi shodhana*. This pranayama is designed to balance the right and left hemispheres of the brain, which in turn brings balance to the central nervous system. This exercise is said to purify the energy channels in the body as well as offer a deep sense of calm. Use it before you have to do a presentation before class, before a job interview, or when you need to release any stress or anxiety you are carrying before bed.

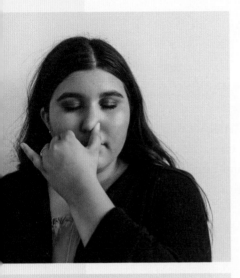

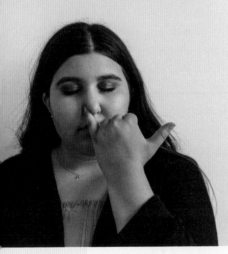

1. Sit tall in a comfortable position.

2. Place your right thumb on your right nostril.

3. Bring your pinky finger to your left nostril.

4. As you inhale, release your thumb and breathe in from your right nostril only for four beats.

5. Plug your nose and hold your breath for one to four beats.

6. Release your pinky finger and breathe out through your left nostril for four beats.

7. Now, breathe in through the left nostril for four beats.

8. Plug your nose and hold your breath for one to four beats.

9. Breathe out through your right nostril for four beats.

10. Try this for ten full rounds.

JOURNAL

A love letter to yourself

For years I have led this letter-writing activity for teens and women on my retreats. It's an exercise that invites you to engage with your soul and listen to your intuition so that you may offer yourself words of wisdom and grace. When the letters are complete, I often pop them in an envelope, seal them, and keep them with me. Then throughout the year I mail them out one by one back to their owners, in hope that my students will open them at a time they need it most. Over the years it has proven to be a beautiful gift. I often write these letters to myself and find them in old journals and it's like, as one teen described it, finding a five-dollar bill in a winter jacket.

Write a letter to yourself from something or someone greater than where you currently stand, like the universe, your ancestors, your angels, or your highest Self. The point is to offer yourself love, words of wisdom, and gentle reminders of who you truly are from a place of tenderness and uncon-ditional respect. There is no wrong way to do this—no one will read your letter unless you want them to.

The below is written by Paloma. I met Paloma when she was fifteen years old. She showed up at my studio one day and never left. She devoted most of her free time to working at the studio in exchange for free yoga classes. She became very dear to me, and I wanted to share some meaningful words she wrote when she was seventeen.

Dear Paloma,

We know you have been scared lately. We have said it once and we will say it again: We are watching over you every day and protecting you.

There is nothing I can stress more than that you need to stay now more than you ever have before. Please do not walk away. Trust us when we say that. We know your legs are tired and your heart is hurting more than ever and it's hurting others, but don't run away. You are here to learn. You need to stay to learn to love and to love yourself.

I am sorry you feel sick right now. I promise you some nights feel worse than others. Every time you step outside, we send a wind to dry your eyes. Every time, my love. Keep looking at the stars and feel small; it's important to know you are simple and the stars are too. They aren't going anywhere, and neither are you.

It breaks our hearts that you can't see the beauty you hold. We see it every day and we are not the only ones. One day you will look into a mirror and love harder than you have ever loved before.

Your mind feels complicated and tangled, but don't listen to it. Please don't listen to it when you don't have any room to think. Things are simple. Find that simplicity and don't let go. Those are the things that matter the most.

Paloma, don't lose sight of how many miles you have walked. They matter and they show. You have a light that can't and won't burn out. You earned beauty and you need to accept it.

So, every bumped hip, every slammed toe, every run to the bus, every quiet night, every doubt, every fight, every tear—we hold your heart tight and make sure you are safe.

We can't promise that it's going to get easier, but we can certainly promise you are going to get better at it.

Let your mind run free and fall, we got you.

Love,

The Universe, forever and always.

YOUR TURN.

the power of
your actions

"The moment
I recognized that
I needed to reintroduce
myself to me was the
moment I understood
that I am the only one
with the keys required
to reach my highest self."

–Sahiti, 18,
NEW YORK CITY, NEW YORK

06

GEMMA

The last day of each retreat, there is one final exercise: each teen is instructed to write a reintroduction letter to their parents, friends, or even the entire world. It's a letter to proudly declare who you are beyond anyone's (including your own) limiting expectations or beliefs about you. It is written with boldness and certainty. It is a chance for everyone to step into the power they have realized within themselves through what they have learned at Girlvana, and share it with the world. It is a way to solidify the new self-discoveries and release the old identities that no longer fit. Once everyone has written their letter, we come back together and, one by one, read our letters out loud.

Gemma raises her hand to read her letter. It is addressed to her mom and dad. Everyone sits attentively, listening with their hearts, which we call *holding space*. Gemma begins to read her profound and eloquent words about who she is becoming and who she has always known herself to be. She speaks to the powerful ways in which she has felt seen, heard, and loved by the group this week. She shares how it has felt to be recognized for who she is and how she no longer feels the need to hide. She speaks about the old identities of who she thought she had to be in order to be loved and accepted. She says that this group has provided her with the space to be fully herself, the most her she has ever been. She smiles and reads that she has never felt free to be herself.

"Mom and Dad," she says, "I'm gay."

As Gemma continues to read her letter, we sit in awe of her deep self-assuredness and relief, beaming at her with pride and admiration. When she finishes reading, we all begin to roar with cheers, tears, and vigorous applause. We leap up for a group hug and smother our Gemma with all the love in the world. Being able to witness someone standing tall and speaking their truth so courageously is the best feeling in the world. The vulnerability met with deep respect and compassion is truly what Girlvana is all about.

A few days later, once everyone has arrived home from the retreat, Gemma shares with us via group text that she has read the letter out loud to her parents. She was able to reintroduce herself to the people that raised her, and let them know who she is and who she is becoming. She was able to find the words to liberate herself and share her truth. And she was met with love and acceptance from her family. To this day, her story is one of my most cherished.

226

In life, we must prioritize our own growth, beyond the expectations of others, in order to be our whole selves.

LETTING GO

The final yama is aparigraha, which is all about letting go of expectations. Gemma's story is a powerful example of someone sharing their truth and letting go of what others might say or think of them. It reminds me of one of my all-time favorite quotes, by Anaïs Nin, a Cuban-French American writer: "And the day came when the risk to remain tight in a bud was more painful than the risk it took to blossom."

You may have already experienced something similar to what this line describes. Has staying small and fitting others' wishes for you become more painful than you can bear? Has releasing others' ideas about you been risky but ultimately worth it? Aparigraha is about exactly this. The other yamas have taught us about self-compassion, speaking our truth, staying present, and feeding our souls—now it is time to let go of who we think we *should* be and step into who we really are, as *we* define it.

Yoga has never been about how flexible you are or how thin you look; it is about getting down to the truth of who you are and celebrating it.

Holding space means listening with your heart.

227

A WINDING PATH

One night it just came to me: *This yoga stuff is working.* I had been changed by it. I was more me than I had ever been.

The path is
winding
but worth it.

The heaviness I had been carrying for years had seemed to disappear. I felt truly met, seen, and loved. I finally had a relationship with myself, one that was kind and truthful and honoring.

The path of self-discovery through yoga can be both tough and tender. Sometimes it gently nudges and other times it smacks us upside the head. And the unfolding process can be really uncomfortable, especially if we are used to numbing out and pretending that we are fine. There will be darkness, but there is also so much lightness waiting on the other side. The journey, though wild, is impossibly rewarding.

As a teen, I had no idea I could feel this good, that I could heal my eating disorder, that I could stop having panic attacks, and that I could be in a relationship that made me feel seen and honored. I had no idea that I had the potential to heal others or change the world. But here I am, just a regular girl with the desire to seek and know myself and ultimately make peace with myself.

Feeling good is possible. It might not always look pretty or be an easy path, but I assure you it is so worth it. I used to have a teacher that would say, "Even if you are walking backwards or in circles on your path, you are still on your path." All of my cumulative struggles have led me here, so I'm grateful for them. Every ex-partner, every failed career endeavor, every body struggle—each one has taught me more about myself so that I could bring Girlvana to the world.

DEAR YOGA

A few years after my first yoga class, I wrote a letter to yoga. When we choose to really see ourselves and bring awareness to our egos and dark thoughts, we can finally begin to heal and find joy. There is no way to bypass it. We have to do the work. But transformation can happen.

Dear Yoga,

I would like to formally thank you for breaking my heart wide open that one fateful night. It was as though you sat in front of me, looked at me dead in the eye, and saw me the way no one else ever had.

I was terrified that the walls I had built around myself would crumble in that instant. But you were soft at the beginning. You removed them brick by brick, just enough to keep me coming back.

Some days you were not as gentle. No, some days you held the sledgehammer in your hands. Some days, you hit my walls harder than others, left me in a pile of rubble, and then asked me, "Who are you now?"

Most days, I would quickly rebuild my barricades and go on playing my well-rehearsed role of perfection. But I would come back to you with my tail between my legs, knowing that I was a fraud.

Just when I thought I had the perfect pair of yoga pants, that I had drunk the right amount of green juice, and that I

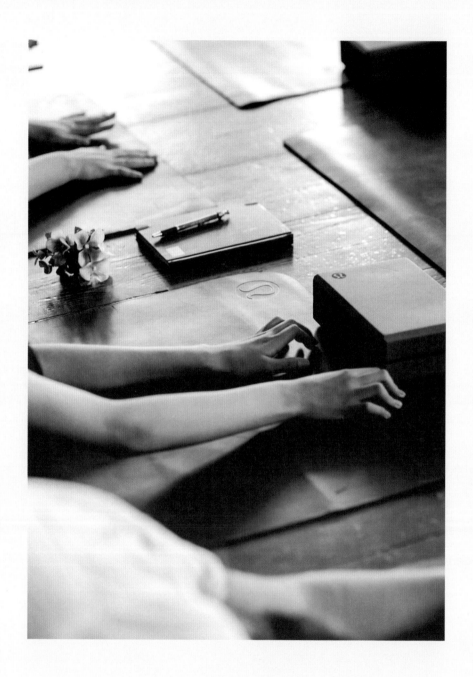

had perfectly batted my eyelashes and folded my hands grace-
fully in prayer, you ripped me from this act and threw me into
the folds of my ugliness, the places I wanted no one ever to see.

And as the sweat poured down my body and the tears slid
down my cheeks, you invited me into a new pose. One that I
was bad at or looked stupid doing, one that made me want to
quit right then and there. You brought me to my knees, Yoga,
but then you took me sweetly into savasana and in my broken
pieces laid out a truth. It was as though it had just hatched,
but you told me it had actually been there all along.

I thought I would be hollow and empty without these
walls, but I was fuller and richer than ever before. I thought I
would be barren and ugly, but I had never felt more beautiful.
You led me into the depths of my own hell, telling me to stay
and bear witness to it.

You said watch.

You said breathe.

You said stay.

I wanted to run so fast and so far but instead I watched
the fire burn. Just like you told me to, Yoga. And when it was
all done, I smudged myself in the ashes and vowed I would
tell everyone that there was a way out of pain. When you laid
me down at the end of each practice, and whispered to me
the answers I have longed for, I felt a love I had never known.
I often wonder how it is that you can continue to hold me in
such a generous presence. I remember that for a long time I
would think, *Am I worthy of this place?*

You tell me *Open, open, open.* And even when I scream *Fuck right off,* you whisper *Gentle, gentle, gentle.* How can you hold me in such roughness? Such resistance? How can you hold all of us hating ourselves and hating you? You don't even flinch. You say, *See you next time.*

You never get offended when people think you're a trend, when we try to brand you or say that you are this and you are that. You just let us come in, soaked in grief and doubt or whatever hell we have created, and you hold us.

You pour honey on our wounds but not before you pour salt. You say we need to feel before we heal. I have really begun to trust you on that one. So much so that I have built a life around you. Told many people about you. Made my dreams come true because of you.

Was it you or was it me all along? Did you break me open so I could free the soul that lay hostage inside, the one shaking with a tape pressed against her mouth, trying to speak? Were you just a catalyst to remove the conditioning and the blocks of pain that clung tightly to my DNA? Were you here all along to show me myself? To hold up the mirror and force me to meet my own eyes—the same way you sat with me that first time?

You said, *This is you. Look at your fullness and the wisdom you possess. Drop your stories and get on with it, girl. There is so much on the other side of this pain. If you get lost, come back, and I will always direct you back home, to free you when you have retreated, to see you when you cannot see yourself, to love you when all love is lost.*

Thank you for seeing the entire universe within me, Yoga. Thank you for not turning away in my darkest hour. Thank you for nudging me into truth. Thank you for peeling back my layers and showing me the way back home.

Love,

xo ally maz

I don't always get it right and neither will you. That is okay. We are human. All that matters is our willingness to come back into alignment with our true nature, our capital-S Self. All I ask is that you feed your heart and not your ego. I ask that you live for you and not for anyone else. I ask that you step into your power. *The world needs you to be you.*

233

YOGA IS POLITICAL

Yoga, as I see it now, is political. There is a reason I want to make teens aware of this practice: I believe that the next generation—your generation—is here to make a massive impact in a way that will help heal the world. I want to equip you with tools I wish I had when I was younger so that you can sidestep some of the tumultuous patterns that were passed down to my generation. Yoga is such a powerful way to bring us back to our true nature so that we don't get swept up in the illusions that this world is trying to sell us in order to keep us small.

Throughout my years of teaching Girlvana, I have come to realize perhaps the most crucial piece of this work: that *to know yourself as a young woman is a political act.* Being who you are is actually an act of resistance. The system is set up so that you, me, and other women like us can run from ourselves and distract ourselves from the truth. And what's the truth? The truth is that we do not need anyone or anything to define us—we hold the power to choose who we are for ourselves. This truth is the opposite of the way the world works right now. In the world right now, the more confused, depressed, and anxious we are, and the more vulnerable we are, the more systems of oppression, like patriarchy and white supremacy, are upheld.

234

To be an unembodied young woman can be a dangerous thing. When we do not have a relationship with the power of our bodies and voices, we can be more malleable for others to take advantage of. And patriarchy benefits from this kind of susceptibility. It's a weakness that can be bought, sold, raped, taken, manipulated, and abused.

I believe that to know yourself is life's greatest pursuit. *Everything* is born out of that place of knowingness. When we do the hard work of getting to know our *yes* and *no*, when we can sense our intuition, when we can face our darkness, when we can calm our anxieties, when we can reset with a deep breath, we strengthen our sense of self. We also become less the target and more the arrow. Imagine if all young women had access to these tools to know themselves. Could the systems that have been in

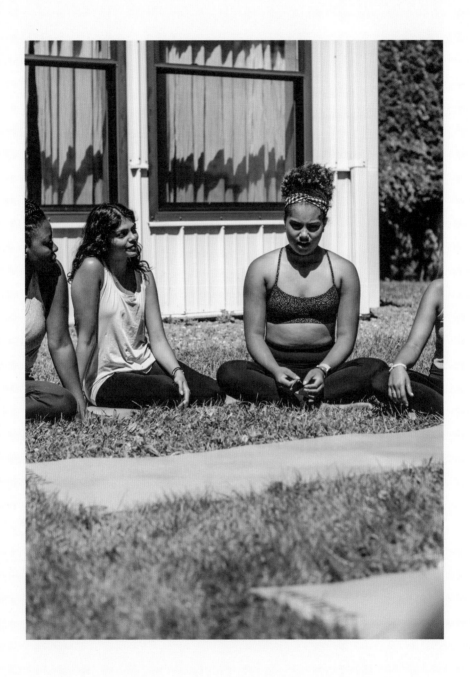

When I rise,
you rise.
When you
rise, I rise.

236

power for centuries handle this new wave of empowered young women? Probably not. It's time for us to work. On my most challenging days, when I can't face myself or the world, I remind myself that showing up is not only for me but for all of us. When I get caught in my own downward spirals of my mind or hung up on how I look or the weight that I am, I am doing a direct disservice to the other young women around me. When you hold certain privileges, you cannot lazily rest in the background of the most pressing world issues. You have to wake up and use what was given to you to carve a deeper and clearer path for your sisters, brothers, and everyone. When I rise, you rise. When you rise, I rise.

When we feel bad, ugly, and unhappy with our bodies, it's important that we realize that we, as females, are not benefiting from these thoughts. In fact, someone else is getting rich off of them. Let's pause on this for a moment. When you feel fat or ugly, and you buy flat-tummy tea and brand-new makeup, someone else is actually benefiting from it. There are companies literally banking on us hating ourselves. Our low self-worth is woven into their marketing strategies so that they can make money and we can stay small. I think of this every time my negative self-talk comes into my mind and threatens to take me down a dark, winding road of "not-enoughness."

We cannot let this continue to happen. Showing up for ourselves can be messy and terrifying, but the other option is to continue to comply with an ancient system that is not set up for our well-being. Try to remember this even on your toughest days.

I used to believe that not liking myself was a secret thing that I would struggle with for the rest of my life. But as I progressed into adolescence it became a bonding tool with other girls, and thus the mindset continued to persist. Once I had a greater understanding of where these thoughts were coming from, I was able to rewire how I thought about myself. I couldn't let anyone benefit from my personal struggles, and when I connected the dots, I started to realize that when I love myself it puts a wrench in that system. When I began teaching Girlvana I was able to see that educating girls on how to love themselves makes an even bigger dent. And when those girls tell their friends, mothers, grandmothers, sisters, teachers, boyfriends, girlfriends, and community— then we can really make an impact.

Instead of telling young girls to smile, be happy, and think positive, I want to help them find the root of these oppressive thoughts they feel. This knowing frees us up from feeling that we are bad, wrong, or messed up. When we are aware, we can start to break this pattern. When we are ourselves and we fully accept who we are, it's a great act of resistance!

We are insanely beautiful, diverse, intelligent, and bold humans in the bodies we were given, showing up and accepting who we are. We are powerfully uplifting ourselves and simultaneously uplifting others. We can be fluid in our gender and sexuality. We can speak up. We can rise. We can be who we are and not have to change or hide.

> If we do not
> help ourselves
> and then help
> others be free,
> no one is
> truly free.

Imagine the possibility of this, and see that this starts with you. Staying silent and complacent in your privilege will mean that other people suffer. Staying absorbed in your own self-hatred means that we, as women, cannot rise. If we can do this work now, we can save the next generation from believing that they are something to be fixed, molded, or changed.

NO VOICE IS TOO SMALL

As we continue to wake up and demand a better world, we must see also that no voice is too small. Sometimes, as I watch the news, I become so overwhelmed by everything that is going on that it almost paralyzes me. In those moments, I ask myself, *What can I even do?*

What I have learned throughout my years of this work is that every single day I must start small, and that it starts with me. My thoughts are a direct reflection of what I see. I see hate, war, racism, sexism—and I also see those things reflected inside of me. When I look deeper and really sit with myself, I know I need to look at where I am at war with myself. I need to see what unconscious biases I am holding. I need to see where as a woman I am quieting myself and holding back. As a white woman I need to look at where I am staying silent and not using my privilege to speak up.

If we can start with what is going on inside of us, then we can bring it to the outside, to the world. It is easy to get caught up in feeling like our voice won't matter (and if you've been paying attention, this is also what we have been conditioned to believe). But speaking up and speaking out is necessary, and never too small of an effort. When I get stuck in my own head about whether what I have to say matters or not, I think of all the women who never get the chance to speak. From social media to music to art, we have so many platforms for expression these days. These are things our ancestors could have never imagined. We need to speak for those who could not. And in looking towards the future, we need to speak so that others who currently can't, will.

So, no, yoga is not about cute poses on a beach or green smoothies and mala beads. It's not about getting flexible or having abs. It is definitely not about being thin or rich or famous. It is about having a voice. It is about ending the cycle of hating ourselves, of being at war with our bodies, of staying quiet and small. It is about no longer hiding who we are for fear of not being liked. Yoga is about being courageous enough to be ourselves. And guess what? We are bringing everyone with us! And I mean everyone, especially the ones who do not look, act, or sound like us. The ones who have different bodies, different abilities, different sexualities, and different backgrounds. We are *all* deserving of this freedom, and we're going to need *all* of us to change the world.

Our silence is a form of violence.

JOINING THE REVOLUTION

Here is a list of things you can do to join this revolution:

- Catch yourself when you are thinking and/or speaking negatively about yourself. Ask yourself, *Who benefits from this?*

- Notice your own unconscious biases around people who don't look like you. When you see microaggressions occurring at your school or in your family, say something. Our silence is a form of violence.

240

- Stand up for other people. Do not stay quiet. In order to disrupt the system, we must use our voices. Call someone out when they are being racist, sexist, homophobic, or transphobic.

A micro-aggression is an indirect, subtle, or uninten-tional act of discrimination against a marginalized group of people.

- Be a good ally. This means using your power and privi-lege to achieve equity and inclusion. Becoming an ally to marginalized communities requires that we actively stand *beside* them versus just "having their backs." Allyship means that we aren't just learning about racism, sexism, homophobia, and transphobia, but we are actively working to dismantle it. Being a good ally takes a lot of listening, so that we know how best to be of service to those different from us.

+ Do not—I repeat, do not—tear another girl down to feel better about yourself. Gossiping, slut shaming, and other mean-girl behavior are products of the patriarchy. This behavior is ancient history and needs to stop. We must transform our friendships and communities, but it starts with us stopping these negative patterns within ourselves and educating others to do the same. Let's have our kids think that being mean to other kids is insanely absurd!

+ If and when you feel ashamed of your body, pause and remember that you, my dear, are not a coincidence. You have stardust coursing through your veins. You have a unique mind, voice, and soul, and *all* of you is undeniably worthy and precious. You are every bit as deserving of love as anyone else. You believing that will change the world.

+ Do not give other people's (ahem, especially boys' or men's) opinions any weight. Someone else's opinions of your body, face, hair, brain, family, religion, or choices do not define you. You get to decide.

+ Share your art with the world, whether it's your poetry, your music, your drawings, or your research. Do not play small.

+ Reject the idea of being popular. There is no such thing as "the popular group." This social hierarchy is a made-up

construct that values privilege and power. What *is* cool
is being kind and compassionate to yourself and others.
If the people you hang out with don't do that, they are
not worth your time.

+ Shave your legs, don't shave your legs, express yourself
through makeup or never wear it. Do whatever makes
you feel good. Do it for you. Do not do it to fit in or to be
liked. Don't do it to adhere to some unrealistic standard.
You are your own statement and you can choose whatever
is right for you. None of it needs to be defined by what
is "ladylike" or "feminine." The new paradigm is here and
you are the captain of defining yourself, not some ancient
gender binary.

+ Start believing that you matter. If you've stopped believing that this is true, here is your reminder. You are not
unworthy or ugly—society is. Together let's rise above
all this BS and create a new world, okay?

This work is ever-evolving and the terms and concepts
will continue to shift and change, but the one thing that will
remain the same is the consciousness. Can we continue to
look inward, to become aware of ourselves and our environment, and to create a safe space within in order to be who we
are? Can we show up for ourselves and can we show up for
others? The answer is yes. I hope this book has shown you

ways to do that. I hope you can see now just how deeply you matter and how deeply we need you. Regardless of what you thought or what you've been told, we don't need you to disappear; we need you to embody all that is you. The world needs you to be you, now more than ever.

Let's serve ourselves and not *the system that got us here.*
Let's serve our spirits and not the beauty industry's standard of what we should look like.
Let's be more than what the world has imagined for us.
Let's be more of what we thought possible.
Let's take up more space in our bodies and more space in the world.
Let's fill ourselves with breath instead of mindless negative thoughts.
Let's be brave enough to accept all the complex and beautiful things that make us who we are.
Let's not look away when oppression or wrongdoing is happening around us.
Let's look within when we are suppressing our own emotions and hurting ourselves.
Together, let's be brave enough to do this work.

THE PRACTICE OF SURRENDER

The last yoga sequence I want to offer is a gentle wind-down, the ending to each yoga flow in the book. On the following page, the last pose in this flow is called savasana. *Savasana* is a Sanskrit word that translates as "corpse pose." It symbolizes the death of the practice.

Just like in nature and in our own lives, death is a recurring theme in the practice of yoga. Death reminds us of the impermanence of all things. It teaches us to appreciate the present moment and shows us how to let go when it is time. In nature, death leads to rebirth—look at winter being followed by spring. Look at the moon. All of this beautiful symbolism shows us that we, too, can have endings and beginnings. We can begin again. Old patterns, bad habits, negative self-talk can die. We can start again. We can be new again.

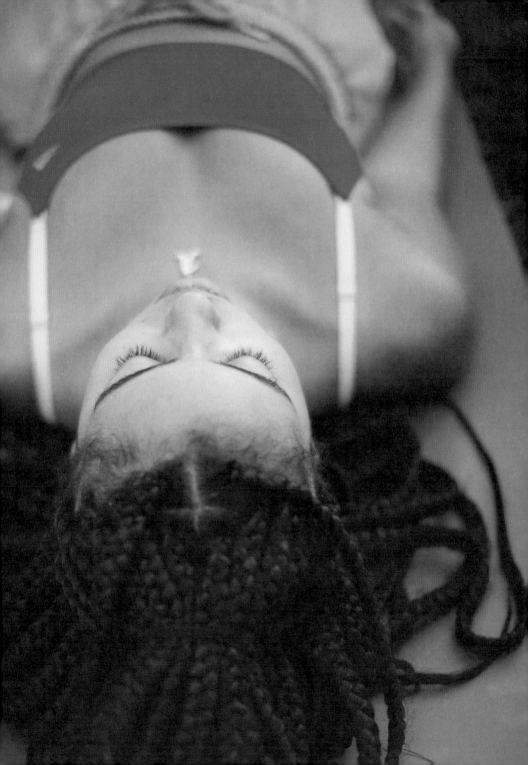

FLOOR FLOW

1. Lying on your back, pull both knees into your chest. Wrap your arms around your knees.

2. Slowly rock from side to side. This movement helps to calm the nervous system, which in turn helps to relax you.

3. Straighten your left leg onto the floor. Continue holding your right knee to your chest for two breaths.

4. Now pull your right knee over to the left and extend your right arm to the right, in line with your shoulder. Turn your head to the right.

5. Hold for five breaths.

6. Repeat on the left side.

7. Release your arms and legs onto the floor.

8. Hold your arms forty-five degrees from your body or resting on your body.

9. Keep your legs hip-width apart or wider, with feet relaxed.

10. Close your eyes and let your body sink into the floor.

11. Stay here for 3 to 20 minutes.

Savasana is an act of surrender. It symbolizes letting go of control, which is especially
helpful if you feel like you are trying too
hard to control every little thing that is
happening in your life. These relaxing poses
can help you soften and surrender the need
to micromanage every aspect of your life.
Think of savasana as your sacred time,
where you don't have to carry or hold on to
the heaviness that you feel. Give yourself
permission to let go and to let what needs
to end, end.

At first, this pose can feel weird or
uncomfortable, but just like with all of
these practices, getting familiar with
being quiet in your body and head takes
time. Be patient and gentle with yourself.

At the closing of each yoga class, we say
the Sanskrit word *Namaste*. When I
first learned the word, it was explained
to me as meaning "the light inside of me
sees the light inside of you." In Girlvana
we expand on this to say, "the light and
darkness inside of me honors the light
and darkness inside of you. I see you in
all of your joy, suffering, beauty, aloneness,
fear, and fortitude. I celebrate all aspects
of you. I bow to everything that you are,
everything you have been, and all that
you are becoming."

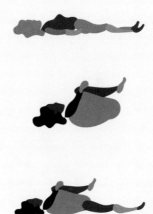

247

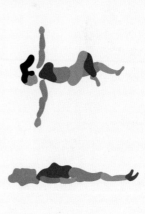

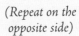

(*Repeat on the
opposite side*)

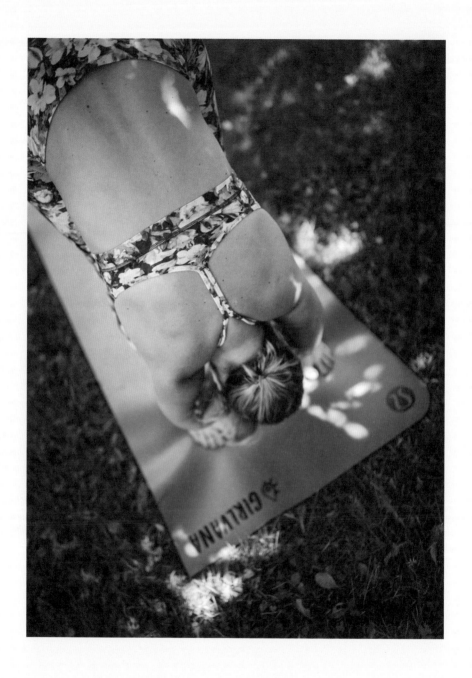

YOU ARE ALREADY IT

This book is not intended to tell you how to feel or what to believe—your connection to yourself and something greater will be defined by you and only you. No one gets to decide that for you. In some cases, we are born into beliefs that are not necessarily our own, and it can be challenging to navigate how we feel about what was pressed upon us. My advice is to keep seeking within. Keep breathing, moving, writing, and finding time to be quiet with yourself. The more we do these things, the more connected we feel.

Yoga means union. The word *yoga* translates from Sanskrit as "to yoke or to bring together." Yoga is the bringing together of the physical, mental, emotional, and spiritual worlds. It is a practice of discovering one's wholeness. You are not broken. You don't need to be fixed. You simply need to tune in to who you already are. You are already it.

MEDITATION TO LET GO

In this meditation we are going to use the power
of visualization and the yama of aparigraha to release
the grip of tension in the head, heart, and body in
order to feel free and spacious.

1. Get comfortable by sitting or lying down.

2. Close your eyes or soften your gaze.

3. Deepen your breath.

4. Notice where you feel tension in your body. See if
   you can direct your breath to where you are feeling
   the gripping in your body.

5. As you inhale, breathe into the tension.

6. As you exhale, imagine it leaving your body.

7. Now imagine, as you inhale, a color of your choosing.
   Let that color fill up your whole body.

8. As you exhale, imagine a black smoke leaving your
   body, and with it any tension or tightness in the body.

9. Repeat this ten times.

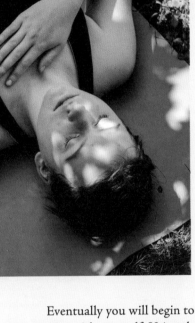

Eventually you will begin to feel more at ease with yourself. Using the visuals of color can help transform the tension in your body to freedom. Ultimately our goal is to feel liberated from tension and negativity in our bodies, minds, hearts, and souls—because you deserve to feel good.

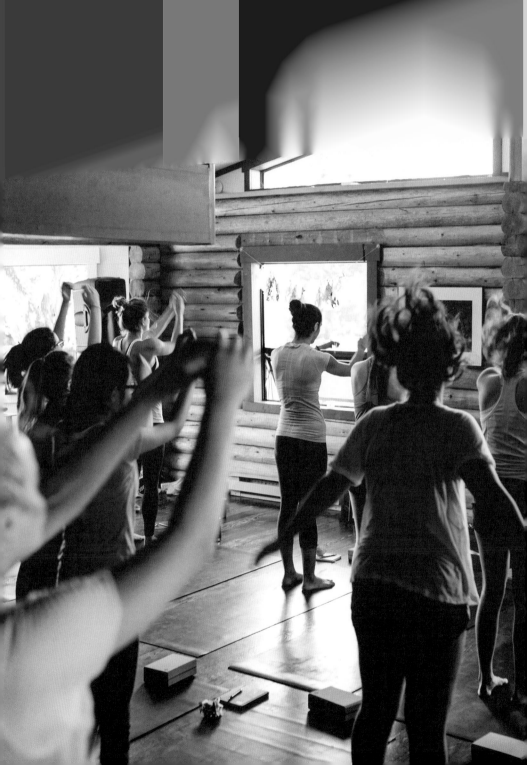

BREATH OF JOY

The last breath exercise I want to teach you is called breath of joy. It is an active breath that invigorates your body, scrubs you clean of stress, and makes you feel alive. This breath is an all-time MVP at Girlvana. It consists of three sharp inhales through the nose and one giant exhale. I like to put on a song and link my movements to the music. It goes like this:

1. Stand tall with a slight bend in your knees.

2. Inhale, swinging your arms in front of you.

3. Inhale, swinging your arms to the side of you (in line with your shoulders).

4. Inhale, swinging your arms over your head.

5. As you throw your arms down, exhale through your mouth with a *ha* sound. As you do this, bend your knees and throw your upper body down toward your knees.

6. Repeat ten times.

Once you finish, stand tall in tadasana and feel the energy this exercise has created. It can feel so freeing to swing your arms around and shout big sounds of *HA!* as you exhale. Once you finish, there is a new energy to behold. A new moment. A new you.

JOURNAL

Your reintroduction letter

I feel like there is no better way to end this book than for you to embark on your reintroduction letter. Now is the time for you to dig deep and spill your heart out on your page to tell the world who you really are. Thinking beyond all conditioning, external expectations, and your own personal "shoulds," write a letter to the world, or to any people of your choosing, and declare who you are!

YOUR TURN.

dear girls

dear girls,

I hate when you hate yourselves. I love when you love your-selves.

When I hear about the advances from men you had to tol-erate, my skin burns like that day it did when I was attacked in my own home. It burns when you speak of the moments you abandoned your own body for another, the times you sliced your skin open just to feel alive, or the moments you stepped on the scale and that number outweighed any sense of self-worth you had.

Dear girls,

I break for you because my own pain still sometimes lives in my own body. I may have put out a lot of those fires, but some-times I can still feel the embers burn.

I don't know more than you—in fact, in many ways, you are much more advanced than I.

Let's keep teaching one another. Let's end the war that we were taught to wage at a young age. Let's stay strong for all the women and girls.

When you want to hurt yourself, please think of me, of us, of all the girls.

When you want to run, stay and feel because in some city, somewhere, there is another girl waking up and recommitting to herself.

As you navigate the next steps of your life, don't forget that you are the answer, you are the one you've been waiting for.

For you. For us. For all the girls,

xo ally maz

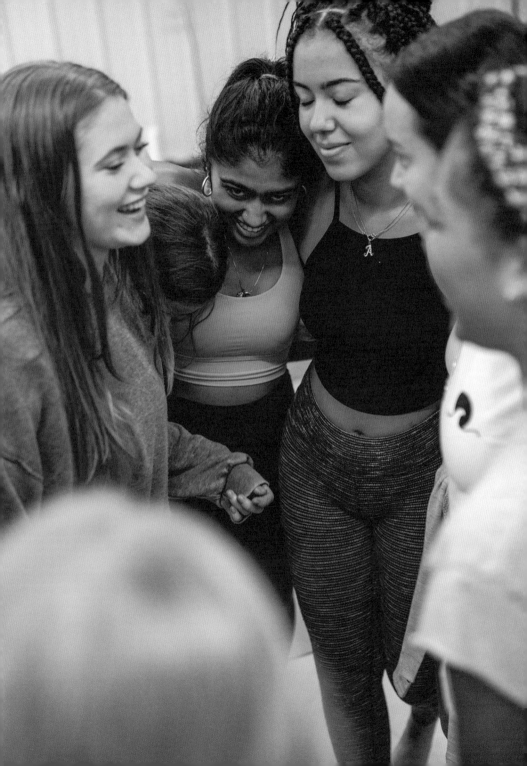

Resources

BOOKS

A list of books that have guided me on my journey, ranging from spirituality, social justice and anti-racism, and creativity.

Spirituality, Yoga, and Wellness

A New Earth by Eckhart Tolle
Breath by James Nestor
Braiding Sweetgrass by Robin Wall Kimmerer
Embrace Yoga's Roots by Susanna Barkataki
Heart Minded by Sarah Blondin
Milk and Honey by Rupi Kaur
The Alchemist by Paulo Coelho
The Body Keeps Score by Bessel van der Kolk, M.D.
The Four Agreements by Don Miguel Ruiz
The Power of Breathwork by Jennifer Patterson
The Untethered Soul Michael A. Singer
The Yamas and Niyamas by Deborah Adele
Women Who Run With the Wolves by Clarissa Pinkola Estés

Social Justice and Anti-Racism

Between the World and Me by Ta-Nehisi Coates
How to be an Antiracist by Ibram X. Kendi
Me and White Supremacy by Layla F. Saad

Sister Outsider by Audre Lorde

Skill in Action by Michelle Cassandra Johnson

Creativity

Big Magic by Elizabeth Gilbert

Bird by Bird by Anne Lamott

The Artist's Way by Julia Cameron

The War of Art by Steven Pressfield

Writing Down the Bones by Natalie Goldberg

WEBSITES

263

A small but important list of websites if you're ever in need of help.

Crisis intervention and suicide prevention services for LGBTQ+

➤ www.thetrevorproject.org

Suicide prevention lifeline

➤ suicidepreventionlifeline.org

Wellness for BIPOC and BIPOC youth

➤ www.naayawellness.com

Vancouver-based eating disorder support

➤ www.lookingglassbc.com

Provides financial assistance to Black women and girls seeking therapy

➤ thelovelandfoundation.org/loveland-therapy-fund

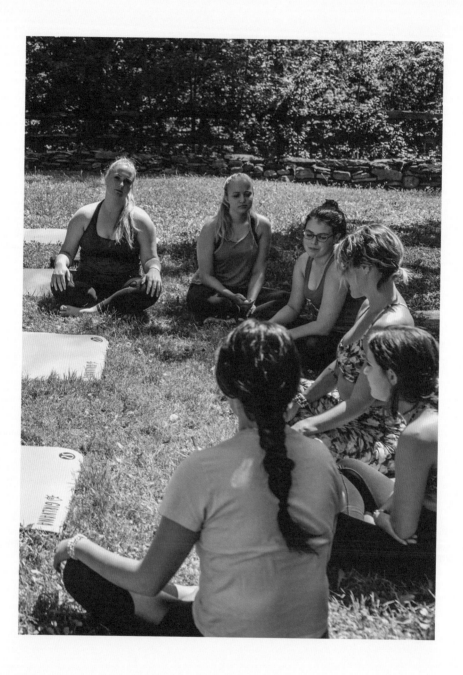

Acknowledgments

I wrote this book all over the world. Most memorable being in the back of a cab in Panama, early jet-lagged mornings in Japan, my parents' house in Vancouver, New York City cafes, and the jungles of Nicaragua. I wrote this book over four years and in that time, I grew and awakened in ways I never expected. This book lived in my heart and in a Word document as my life took new forms in new cities, with new people and new experiences. Throughout this time, one thing remained: the desire for this book to come to life. It was always on my mind. It was always with me.

This book would not have been possible without the following humans.

To my editor, mentor, friend, Bhavna, you are a true teacher and like a true teacher, you did not give me the answers when I was in need, you simply guided me back to myself to find them within. Thank you for your belief, trust, care, vision, perspective, and love. I am awestruck by the depth of this relationship. There is no Girlvana without you.

Mom, this book is born of your own flesh, bones, and blood. This work is yours just as much as it is mine.

Dad, thank you for telling me it was always possible. Because of you, so much of the unimaginable has been born.

To my brother, Zack, if every man showed up the way you do, I am certain that world would be a much better place. I love you and I love Jenn and Olive.

To my husband, Bill. You were a constant force encouraging me to keep going when I didn't think I could.

Jian, you know.

To my mentors, Jess, Ash, Maddy, Boz, you are infinite space holders. Bad boys for life. Thank you for the tireless years of guidance, laughter, and unwavering support. Your friendship is the backbone of Girlvana.

To every single mentor who has graced these retreats with compassion, love, education, and care, thank you. Jessie Hutton Nelson, Sashah Rahemtulla, Adriana Koc-Spadaro, Megan Lawson, Rachel Ricketts, Carolyn Budgell, Bree Melanson, Sarah Blondin, Jacqueline Jennings, Lisa Bay, Emma Collins, Thea Gow-Jarrett, Justine Sones, Sinikiwe Dhliwayo.

To my teachers, Shakti, Clara, Christine, Meghan, Sjanie, Chris, and Georgina, thank you for your teachings and holding me with grace as I found my way.

To Roda, thank you for teaching me how to move through resistance and being my constant cheerleader through this process.

To Nico, Ali, Mel, Cat, your care, organization, and creativity gave Girlvana the legs to run and run far. Thank you for creating structure, keeping faith, and holding me together.

To Abdi, Rachel, Kate, and the entire Appetite team, thank you for your hard work and dedication to this project.

To Gabby Bernstein, thank you for believing in this book.

To my Lululemon family, thank you for your support and encouragement over the last decade. So much was made possible because of it.

To Zach and Ryan, thank you for introducing me to Robert. That coffee meeting changed my life. Robert, thank you for trusting my vision.

To my teachers who have gone on to spread the Girlvana message all over the globe, thank you for sharing the magic. The young people of this world need you. Thank you for showing up for them.

To all my girls—yes, you. The very ones that showed up each day. The ones that breathed together, cried together, laughed together, grew together. Your bravery and vulnerability have defined my life. I undoubtedly know that I was put on this planet for this very purpose—to know you, to love you, to see you flourish. Thank you for trusting me.

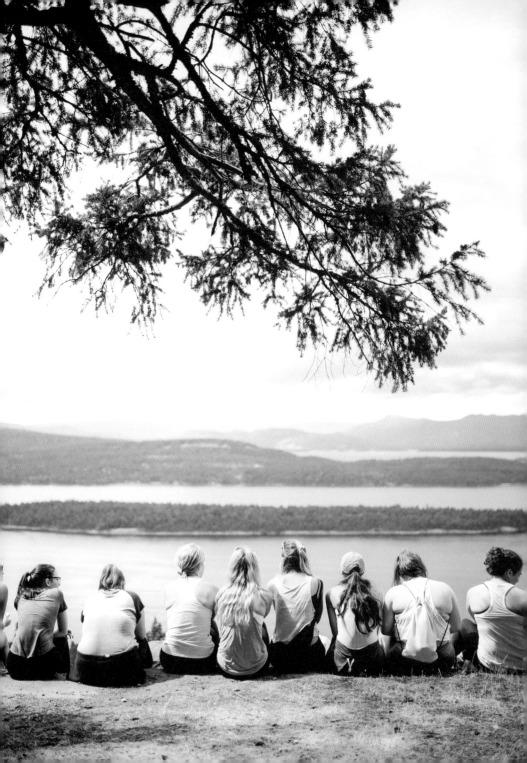

Index

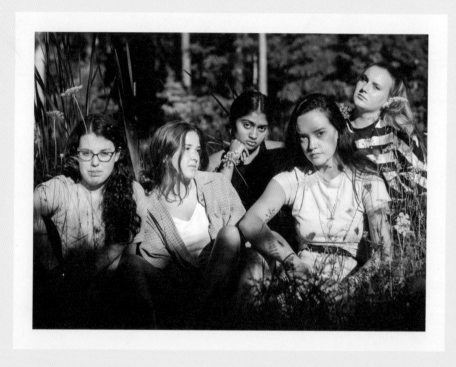